Earth Healing with the Nature Angels & Elemental Masters

Sarah Hunt

DEDICATION

To the angels and elementals with heartfelt thanks and love for their
inspiration and guidance.

CONTENTS

ACKNOWLEDGMENTS

To my friend Jo for her messages of inspiration and her absolute belief in my abilities with all my spiritual work.

INTRODUCTION

I was inspired a couple of years ago to put together two workshops connecting people to the Nature Angels and elementals. I had connected with the Nature Angels who explained the importance of us helping Mother Earth to heal. They explained to me that part of the way that we can help Mother Earth is to spend time healing ourselves, for we cannot heal others unless we are willing to heal ourselves. They reminded me again of the importance of working with the spiritual laws and that the message they want to bring to those of us on Earth is one of peace and love.

Having done a lot of reading around the subject of Atlantis and other spiritual times and whilst looking around me at the world that we live in today it is very apparent that sadly man has moved away from a spiritual way of living and as a result of this has abused the Earth by taking from her continually and not being prepared to give anything back. As man has become more and more materialistic, he has taken more and more from Mother Earth and does not seem to realise that his actions have caused pain and will deplete the natural resources available to us. This situation cannot be allowed to continue as it is detrimental to the health and well-being of Mother Earth and all of us who reside on her.

Gaia has decreed that Mother Earth will ascend and so it will be. In order for this to happen Mother Earth needs to heal and she is going through some major shifts at the moment as she cleanses herself of all the negativity that mankind has created on and in her. As she rebirths we will see changes in the weather and more 'natural disasters' as she clears the negativity and karmic debt that man has built up.

The ley lines need to be cleared so that energy can flow through them again freely as do the waters of the world. The crystal grids are changing as they are cleared and reformed in the formation that is required now as Earth lifts her vibration.

There is a lot of work for us to do but remember that mankind has created the mess and so it is not just the Earth that needs healing but man himself and we can help with this by working on ourselves and healing our own issues as well as healing others. This way we will lift our vibration and so be able to hold more light in our energy systems. As we shine more light into the world and indeed the universe we will be assisting Mother Earth with her healing too.

In this book you will meet some new angels, (who were brought to us by Diana Cooper in her book A New Light on Angels), who have come to Earth to assist with the cleansing process and to help lift Earth's vibration.

You will also meet the Elemental Masters and some of the different elementals themselves who all have different roles, each one as important as the next, as we move through the ascension process and into the fifth dimension.

The following messages from the angels give some insight as to how we may be able to help. I will also include some meditations so that you can work with different groups of these beautiful beings of light and assist them with the healing of Mother Earth that needs to take place. They will also help you to heal yourself as well.

It is with great love that we are with you today for we know how you love the Earth and wish to be of assistance during this time of ascension. There is much work to be done to assist Mother Earth as she rebirths and moves into a new dimension. Man has done much damage over eons of time and has lost sight of the knowledge that he needs to work in harmony with Mother Earth and all who live on her. His need for control and power and his greed have caused many problems for Mother Earth. The abuse of your planet must stop. It is time for all beings to live in harmony once more with Mother Earth for you all came from the same source and are all one with each other and with Source.

We will work closely with you for the good of all and will guide you onto your soul path so that your soul purpose is completed for your current incarnation. There are many different ways that you can help Mother Earth, so be open to new ways of thinking and new opportunities to assist her and all those who reside on her.

There will be more natural disasters as you call them and you will notice changes in your weather systems. These are all part of the cleansing system and part of what is needed in order for Mother Earth to ascend. Lady Gaia has decreed that Earth will ascend to the fifth dimension and so it must be.

There are many battles taking place both on Earth and within the Etheric Realms between light and dark. It is time for light to shine and fill even the darkest corners of the universe for darkness is just an illusion and may be filled with light. We must work together to overcome the darkness so that the Earth is filled with love and light and so that peace and happiness may reign once more on planet Earth.

There are many new energies that have been coming into the Earth and will continue to be poured in. This is to enable the ascension of your planet and all those who reside on her. Many do not understand what is happening to them and may find themselves feeling lost and confused as the energetic shifts take place. We ask you to surround them in love and light so that they may come to understand the changes that are taking place.

There are many who have agreed to help cleanse the planet by passing during a 'natural disaster' taking with them some of the karma so that it can be transmuted in the higher realms. We ask that you send out love and light to them when these situations occur so that they may heal more quickly and come to an understanding of the great work that they have done when they pass.

Remember that your world is a mirror and is reflecting back to you that which needs healing in you. To assist Earth healing and raising the consciousness of the planet it is as important to look within and heal your own issues as well as assist with healing others and the Earth.

You do not need to be working with nature or animals on a physical level to be able to help us. You may wish to make your contribution by tending your garden lovingly, growing your own produce, picking up litter or gently placing a spider outside.

As you connect with us notice how your connection with nature and the natural world increases. See how you are connected and how much brighter and lighter everything looks. Take the time to be in the present moment and notice the beauty around you for you live in a beautiful world filled with precious moments if only you will step back and allow yourself to look.

Become aware of the elementals who will assist you with working with Mother Earth and her kingdoms if you ask them. We must all work together to raise the vibration and consciousness of mankind. For when man finds peace, love and happiness within, so shall there be peace, love and happiness on Earth.
We love and honour you and thank you for working with us.'

Channelled by Sarah Hunt 31/7/12

3

It is with great love that we are here with you tonight for there has been much progress. The vibration of Earth is far higher than was expected to be at this point and we are pleased to see how many lightworkers are awakening and assisting with the healing process that must take place for Mother Earth to continue to ascend. There have been many events which have helped to raise the vibration on Earth and this has allowed new higher vibration energies to come into the Earth Plane. A portal of light was opened as a result of the energies which came in between the 8th and 23rd October 2014. The lunar eclipse and the solar eclipses enabled more light to be brought in to assist the Earth with her rebirth and healing process.

There has been much upheaval as Mother Earth clears the negativity that man has created. The ensuing chaos as the old energies are released may be lessened by the assistance of light workers. More light and love needs to be sent to Mother Earth to assist her with transmuting the old negative energies and to release the karma that has been accrued by man's abuse of her and her resources.

It is time for man to understand that he must work in harmony with Mother Earth and that there must now be a balance of energies. Man cannot continue to take from Mother Earth without giving back to her in some way.

Man must come to understand the spiritual laws so that he understands how to work in harmony with the universe and the Earth. He must start to recognise his many blessings and be thankful for them. He must move back into a more spiritual way of being so that once again he becomes connected with all that is. Once again he will come to realise that we are all one and are all here to lift our vibrations in order to ascend with Mother Earth.

There are many that resist and have not yet awoken to their true selves. They will be cajoled and encouraged to open their eyes to their true spirit, their very soul. For light will penetrate even the darkest corners of the universe and love will dissolve the most negative of energies.

There is to be no escape, Earth is ascending and has been for some time and those who reside on her must ascend too, unless they have agreed to leave the planet in order to release some of the karma that man has created. As they heal in spirit, they too will ascend as they move forward on their path.

We the Angels of Nature and elementals wish to work with you all in order to continue to assist the process of healing and ascension that is our path and the path of many who will follow us. Earth will ascend for it has been decreed by Gaia and so it must be.'

Channelled by Sarah Hunt 4/11/14

So as we can see the Nature Angels and elementals want to work with us to help Mother Earth to heal for they are the nature spirits and are closely connected with her and her needs and can therefore guide us with the healing help that she requires. They also want to assist us with our own healing and indeed healing ourselves is key if we are to be able to lift our vibration and ascend as well.

I feel sure that as we work more and more closely with these beautiful beings we will learn a great deal not only about the Earth but about ourselves too.

We are very blessed to be living on Earth at this time as we are in a position to be able to really make a difference to Mother Earth especially on a spiritual level, for without her we would not be able to learn the lessons we have come to learn or understand our emotions or our sexuality. Earth is indeed a very special school of learning within our wonderful universe and this is an opportunity for us to really connect with her once more as we learn to work in harmony with her for the greatest good of all. Earth teaches us about ourselves. Mirroring things about us that we do and don't like so that we come to understand the deepest recesses of our soul.

It is also important to understand the laws of the universe as this will help us when working with the angels and elementals and will help us to go with the flow rather than fight our way uphill through our life.

The meditations, healing images and messages within this book will connect you with the elemental beings (i.e. the fairies, sylphs, salamanders and many others) angels, (such as Ariel, Purlimiek, and Buytylil,) the Elemental Masters and Gaia herself.

May your connection with these beings become an established one where you can work with them for the greatest good of all.

5

WORKING WITH THE HEALING ENERGY IMAGES

Each of the angels and Elemental Masters that you will meet in this book has channelled a healing energy image through me which you can work with in meditation to assist you with your own personal healing. You may also like to ask the being of light to send the energies from their image out to Mother Earth to assist her with her healing too.

Each image emits the energies of divine love and healing through the image, colours and shapes, which if you are sensitive you will be able to feel as soon as you connect with the picture.

To work with an image in meditation, ensure that you have cleared the space you are going to meditate in of any negativity. You may wish to do this by using tingshas (Tibetan symbols), a singing bowl, incense or smudging with white sage whilst asking from the heart that all negative energies be transmuted to love and healing and sent back from whence they came. Alternatively you may prefer to just send a thought out to the Angelic Realm asking them to clear the energies for you whilst thanking them for doing it, trusting that it will be done.

You may wish to have some relaxing music playing in the back ground and some incense or a scented candle burning, but please ensure that if you are burning incense or a candle that it is in a safe place where it can't be knocked over and ensure that it is extinguished once you have finished.

Choose an image that you wish to work with in meditation and then put some protection around yourself. You may wish to surround yourself in a bubble of protective light or to simply ask Archangel Michael to put his cloak of protection around you.

Ensure that you are sitting in a comfortable position so that you can focus on the image and then allow yourself to just gaze at it. Let your eyes relax so that you feel as if you are looking through it. Keep your gaze on the image for at least five to ten minutes or as long as you feel you need to be there. You may also find yourself wanting to close your eyes and stay in a meditative state holding the image in your mind's eye.

You may become aware of the image changing shape, or you may feel as if you have merged with it. You may also get messages in the form of pictures, words or images. Just go with the flow and allow the image and being of light to communicate with you in whatever way they need to. (It might be useful to have a pen and pad handy so that you can jot down any information that you have received.)

As you meditate on the image you may also become aware of the healing energies moving into your energy system from it. You might experience, tingling, warmth or a feeling of cold in particular areas of your body or you may feel very relaxed. Just allow these energies to come to you as they will assist you with your own personal healing.

When you feel ready to bring yourself back, take a few deep breaths and wiggle your toes and fingers so that you bring your awareness back to your body and the room. Then imagine, feel or see roots growing out of your feet down into the centre of Mother Earth and wrap them around the large amethyst crystal that is there so that you are completely grounded. Thank the image and being of light for working with you and remember to be thankful for the healing and protection that you have also received.

You may wish to work with the same image for several meditation sessions or you may find yourself drawn to a different one each time. Let your intuition guide you as your higher self knows what is needed and what is for your highest good.

Each of the images for each being of light in this book is a healing energy image for you to meditate on.

THE IMPORTANCE OF SELF-HEALING

Whilst this book is about healing Mother Earth and working with the Nature Angels, Gaia and the elementals to achieve this, it is important to understand the need for self-healing.

The spiritual laws are important to understand as well, as they will enable us to grow on many levels if we work with them with the right intent and with love.

Our bodies have important feedback mechanisms that teach us about ourselves. We have forgotten how to listen to our bodies and continue to store negative emotions within them, which in turn may lead to us manifesting a physical or mental dis-ease. I use the word dis-ease like this as when something is not right, our body is at 'dis-ease' with itself.

Those of you who are attuned to Reiki or work with crystals or do any other form of healing where you are working with energy in some way, will already have some understanding of how we have an energetic body as well as a physical body. There is a need to keep it all in balance, which you may wish to do with therapies such as Reiki, spiritual healing, crystal healing or acupuncture, to name a few. Those of you who aren't familiar with this kind of healing may find it a useful subject to look into.

Healing work may also be done in meditation with the assistance of the angels, elementals, your guides, Ascended Masters and indeed any other being of light.

For you to start healing yourself it is useful to look at a few of the spiritual laws.

The Law of Healing:

Healing occurs because love and light transmute the lower vibrations of dis-ease.

Everything is light and light is energy. Your physical body is built by the energy of your consciousness not only from your current life but over many lifetimes. If each soul only had one life it would be unfair for one person to be healthy whilst another had physical limitations. You are on Earth to

8

experience life in a physical body and certain physical choices will have been made prior to your birth which may appear as physical limitations. Your personality then makes choices moment by moment which will affect your health and well-being.

There are two basic emotions on Earth. One is love the other is fear.

When you resist and refuse to acknowledge your spiritual self your chosen experiences come from a place of fear. You then create blocks in your energy system in the form of negative emotions, thought and behaviour patterns, which if not released may then manifest into physical or mental dis-ease. When you refuse to acknowledge your spiritual self you cut off the divine energy supply and your physical body starts to deteriorate.

When you are happy and flowing with love the cells in your body respond by being healthy; as love is a high frequency energy which keeps the energy pathways in your body flowing.

Negative emotions such as anger, rage, jealousy, and guilt block that flow of loving energy as they are low vibration energies. When healing, which is a high vibration energy, takes place these negative blocks are lifted out so that your energy can flow again properly.

You must ask permission before giving anyone healing, but it doesn't matter whether you ask the person directly or you ask their higher self. For healing to take place the person concerned must want to be healed. The principle is the same for animals, plants and the Earth too. You must ask them if they would like healing.

When you are working with someone's energy you are entering a very private space. Think of it as going to someone's house. You wouldn't go in without having first knocked and then been invited in.

For some, the disease may be teaching them something, and is often their karma, so you would not be serving them and their growth by healing it. For others it may not be the right time for them to heal and as a Reiki healer I always allow people to come to me when the time is right for them. They may have expressed at an event that they wish to come and see me for healing and if they don't want to make an appointment there and then I never push them as I know they will come to me when the time is right for them and they are ready to heal. It may also be that they have a spiritual contract with someone else to heal them and they haven't connected with that person yet.

9

If you want someone to heal then you are attached and need to cut the energetic cords between you to allow them to make their own decisions. We do not have the right to decide what is for the other person's highest good.

If the person is too young or too ill to give you an answer then you must ask their higher self. When you do this you will sense whether it is the right thing to do or not and if the answer is no then do not send or give them healing.

Healing is a very powerful frequency and if you impose healing on someone and heal their disease when they do not wish you to do this, you will have to bear the karma of that disease in this lifetime or another. It is therefore important to use your intuition. Healing will flow through you automatically if the situation and time is right.

The same goes for Mother Earth; you must ask her if she would like you to send her healing. Listen to what she has to say as she may ask you to do something very specific to assist her.

The Law of Request:

The universe, Angels, Elementals, and other beings of light are waiting to help you. All you need to do is ask.

Under Universal Law you must ask for help if you want it and you must allow others to ask for your help if they want it rather than bowl in and rescue them. If you are too quick to help someone who hasn't asked for help then you may prevent the person from sorting the situation out themselves and learning the lesson they were meant to learn. Your help is likely to be unappreciated or even ignored and if you force your help onto someone you will bear the karma if it goes wrong.

If however, someone is in danger then of course you must step in and help them. If you are upset by the mess someone else is in then it is an indication that you need to look at yourself rather than rescue the other person.

Remember that the other person will ask for help when they are ready to and until that time you need to look at what they are mirroring to you, so that you can heal that in yourself.

You would not want anyone to jump in and sort things out for you if you had a difficult situation to deal with, as you would probably see it as them trying to interfere.

In the spiritual realm no divine being, whether they are a guide, angel or other being of light would dream of interfering in your life, although they will step in to prevent an accident if it is not something you need to experience and they will save you from death if it is not your time to go.

Divine beings will stand and watch you with compassion and love, if making a mess of a situation is what is required for you to grow spiritually. It would not only be bad manners for them to interfere but it would also stop you from growing, learning and becoming stronger.

There are times when it is appropriate to ask for help but this needs to be done in a calm way with strength rather than by shouting the odds and demanding the help.

Those of you on a spiritual path will know that you need to go within to find the answers as we all have inner wisdom and knowledge. As soon as you are ready for what you need to know or learn the teacher will appear. So, when you are ready to formulate the question from a place of calm centredness you are ready to know the answer. The answer may come from another person, a book, a programme on the television or a radio programme, for example.

When you feel that you want help, you need to be very clear on exactly what help it is that you want. Meditate on what it is you want first and then ask the angels, elementals or your guides (or whichever beings of light you wish to address) for the help that you require. They will always help you.

Equally if you wish to assist with healing someone or Mother Earth then you must ask them if they would like your help.

The Law of Gratitude:

Gratitude brings many more blessings to you so count your blessings and be grateful for them and watch them multiply.

This is one of the most important laws of the universe and means giving thanks from the heart. When you do this, energy flows from the heart bringing wonderful responses from other people and the universe. If you pay lip service to gratitude or feel you 'ought' to say thank you, then you get a very different response.

When you are totally grateful to someone for something they have done they feel the energy of the thank you and want to give more to you. Equally when you send out heartfelt thanks to the universe for all the blessings in your life the universe responds by sending you more blessings. This is the same for the angels, elementals and any other beings of light.

Appreciating the world around us is important so when you see a beautiful sunrise or sunset or a beautiful butterfly or smell the fragrance of a beautiful flower remember to say thank you to Gaia and the Nature angels and elementals.

When you appreciate people and show them this by saying thank you, you will find that behaviour towards you will change in a positive way. If we want to change things around us then we need to look at ourselves first. Take the time to appreciate yourself and the gifts that you have as it will empower you to move forward on your path and bring more positive experiences to you.

Remember too that within every challenging situation there is the gift of a lesson which we need to appreciate and give thanks for.
Learning to be more appreciative of not only the people around you, but the world around you as well, will make you feel happier and more at peace as well as having a positive impact on others. As you start to say thank you for all your blessings to the universe, even for the smallest of things you will find more positive blessings coming your way.

The angels and all other divine beings like to feel appreciated too, so when you have asked them for help remember to thank them as soon as you have put the request in, and when what you have asked for comes about. They will then help you more and more and your life will flow with positive things and happiness.

We, as humans are truly blessed, but we need to acknowledge this and give thanks. So remember to be positive and appreciate and look for the good in every person and situation. Give praise generously and be loving and kind. Celebrate life and your own magnificence and be happy so that you radiate light out into the world.

NATURE ANGELS

There are four main angels which I am going to introduce to you in this chapter. They are Archangels Ariel, Purlimiek, Butyalil and Gersisa. These Angels will work with you for the good of the Earth, and the nature and animal kingdoms. They will also connect you more deeply with the elementals. Purlimiek, Butyalil and Gersisa are new angels to Earth who have come to assist with the ascension process.

Archangel Ariel

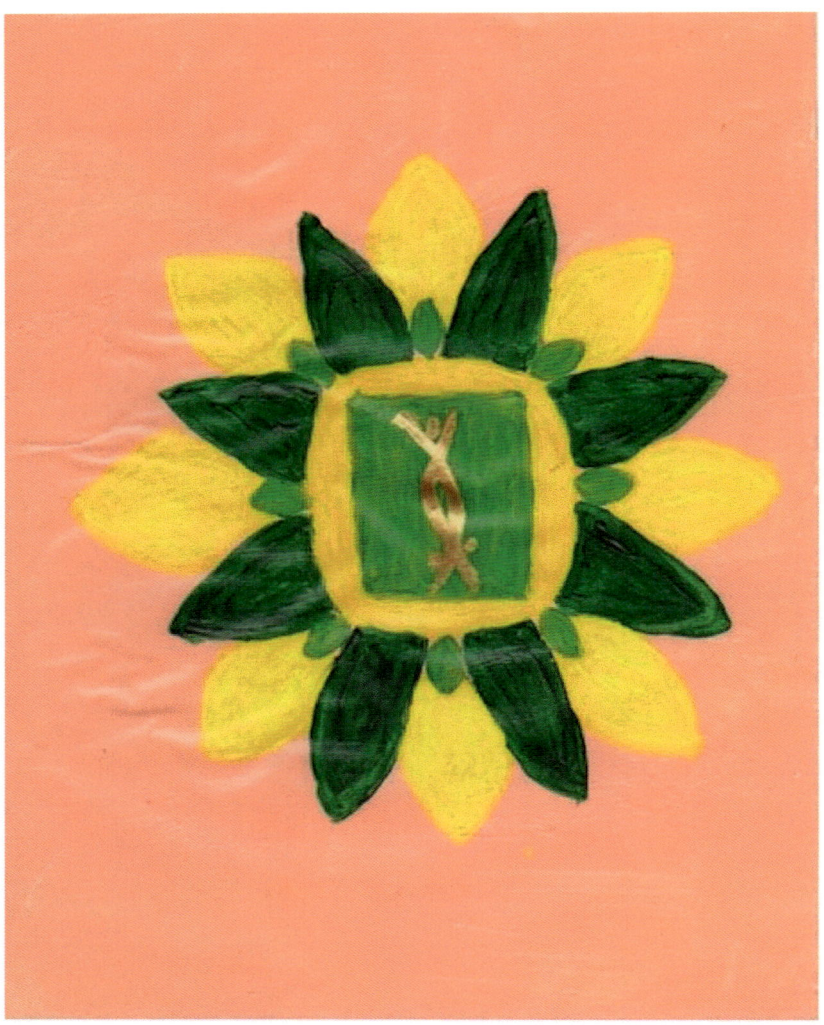

The meaning of Ariel's name is 'Lion or lioness of God' and so this Archangel is often seen depicted with a lion's head. As you connect with Ariel you may become drawn to lions in some way or see visions of them. Ariel is also associated with the wind so you may feel a breeze around you when Ariel is close by.

Ariel works closely with King Solomon assisting with manifestation, spirit release (also known as rescue work - please be aware that this is specialised work and should never be done on your own or without an experienced medium) and Divine magic (magic is often seen as something that those not working for the light do however magic may be used for the light with the right intentions).

Ariel oversees the sprites which are the nature spirits associated with water. They are similar to fairies and their purpose is to maintain healthy environments close to water (such as oceans, lakes, rivers, streams and ponds). Ariel will ask you to work with her as her mission is to purify and protect the water environments and their inhabitants. As you work with her you may be rewarded with wonderful manifestations and increased powers. Ariel is also involved with healing and protecting nature which includes the nature and animal kingdoms especially the wild ones. If you find an animal that is hurt call upon Ariel to assist with the creatures healing.

Dear one I am concerned with the planet that you live on and am working to assist the cleansing and purifying of it. I request your assistance with this and will work with you to guide you as to how you may help me and the elementals in achieving this.

There is so much pollution that has been dumped into the waters of the Earth and it is greatly affecting the inhabitants of the waters and surrounding land. Man has become so ignorant that he does not have any concern about how dumping his waste will affect the flora and fauna of the planet. Man thinks he can harness Mother Earth but this is not possible and Mother Earth is making it clear that she will no longer tolerate such arrogance and lack of consideration for the other earthly inhabitants.

Together we can make a difference in clearing the waters of the Earth of all the negativity but you do not need to reside close to the waters to make a difference. There is so much that we can do together on an energetic level that will assist Mother Earth with her cleansing and re-birthing process.

I am responsible for the elementals in particular the sprites who oversee the waters of the planet. They too will work with you to assist with the cleansing of the planet. These elementals are working hard to cleanse the waterways but man needs to realise that he must take responsibility for his actions and the damage that he has caused. He needs to be re-educated so that he understands that he must work in harmony with the planet so that he no longer causes any damage to her.

There is no need for all the damage that is being done to the planet for you have the technology that is required to use the Earth's resources in a more balanced way but man in his greed wishes to use all the Earth's resources and without any consideration for the consequences or the needs of Mother Earth. This can no longer be. Greed and power are qualities of the over active Ego and this is changing, for the new energies that have come into your planet are aligning ego with the spiritual bodies, but there are still those who will resist this alignment and will continue in their destructive ways. If they do not start to learn they will find that the earth's resources will soon run out and then they will have to look at other ways of providing power and transport.

I also work with the sylphs who are overseen by Dom. The sylphs work with the wind to cleanse Mother Earth. When the winds are high and strong connect with the sylphs and ask them to be more gentle as they cleanse the air. Send out love and light to assist with the cleansing process so that there is no need for such strong winds to blow. For when they are strong it is because there is a need for a lot of cleansing to take place.

There is much to be done as you move towards the Age of Aquarius. As you connect with me I will guide you and assist you and I will give you the energy and inspiration that you need to be able to do this work.
I love you and honour you and thank you for working with me.'

Channelled by Sarah Hunt 31/7/12

Archangel Purlimiek

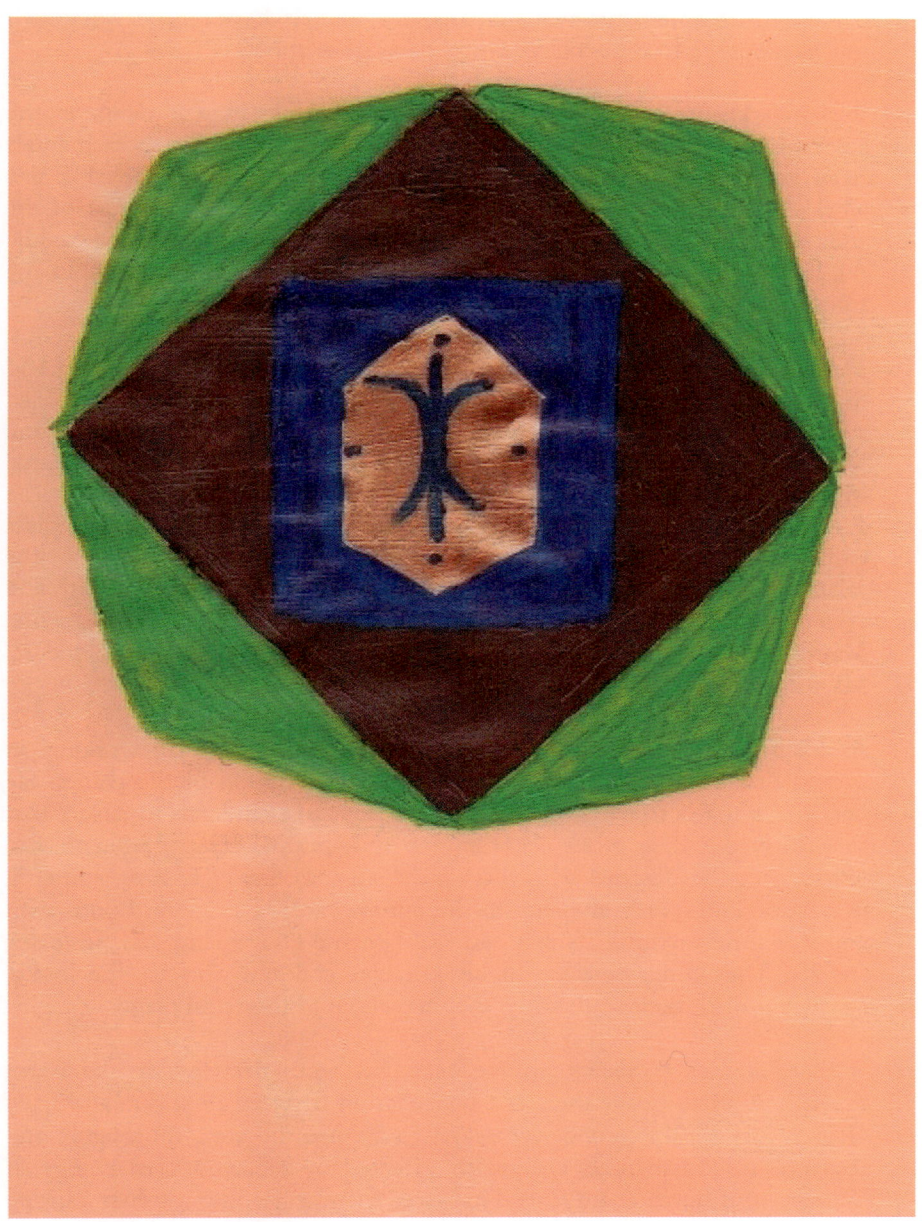

Archangel Purlimiek is in charge of the Nature Kingdom and the elementals which are nature spirits who are called Elementals because they do not contain all the elements that humans and animals have, Some work with one element whilst others have more than one element.

Purlimiek ensures that they are all working together in accordance to the spiritual laws for the highest good of Earth. He has invited new elementals from another universe to assist with the cleansing of the planet. He also works with Archangel Butyalil who is the Cosmic Angel in charge of the stars and energies around the Earth, Archangel Gersisa, the angel of Middle (Hollow) Earth who looks after the ley lines and movements within the Earth and Archangel Fhelyai who is in charge of the Animal Kingdom.

Purlimiek works with the Great Master of Poseidon who is planning and managing the cleansing process. If some form of purification is needed such as a hurricane, storm or earthquake they call upon the Elemental Master who commands his elements to take action. Dom is the Elemental Master of air and will order the sylphs to raise the wind, Neptune is the Elemental Master of water and he will tell the mermaids, sprites and kyphils to move the waters. Thor is the Elemental Master of fire and he tells the salamanders to fan fire and Merlin is the Elemental Master of the Earth and asks the pixies, elves and gnomes to move the Earth. Taia is the Elemental Master of Middle (Hollow) Earth and works with the other Elemental Masters from Middle Earth.

Archangel Purlimiek ensures that the elementals are all working in accordance with the spiritual laws for the highest good of the planet. He designates angels to oversee each of the groups of elementals to ensure that they carry out their work according to the spiritual laws. Purlimiek also works with the dragons who offer great wisdom, courage, love, strength, protection and companionship to the human race. If a dragon bonds with you it will never break its link and will become your friend and protector for life. They often befriend highly sensitive children who are fun loving and will protect their souls when they travel out to the astral planes at night.

If there is a deep need to move negativity from deep within the Earth through an earth quake there is a consultation between Poseidon and Lady Gaia before the elementals are asked to cleanse the area, thoroughly and respectfully. Elementals are greatly affected by the emotional energy of humans so if humans are fearful it causes them to go into a frenzy causing greater damage. It is therefore helpful for us to send out love and light to any areas that are being cleansed to help bring peace and calm back to the area.

When you see something beautiful in nature remember to thank Archangel Purlimiek.

'I am Purlimiek and it is great love that I come to you today. I am indeed new to planet Earth but I am not new to the universe. I am here to oversee and guide the Elemental Kingdom in order to assist Gaia with the cleansing process which must take place for her to be able to ascend. It is important that man learns not to fear the elementals and the work they do, but rather work with them to assist the ascension process. As you connect with me, I will enable you to connect with the elementals more closely, so that we can all work for the greater good of Earth and all who reside on her.

We must work together to bring more understanding to man of the importance of showing respect love and kindness to all who reside in the Nature Kingdom, as animal, vegetable and mineral. For as we work in harmony with each other we can achieve great things. Every living thing has a part to play on planet Earth and there needs to be more balance between man and nature. The Nature Kingdom is not a kingdom to be controlled and dominated by mankind but connected with and harmonised with so that all living things may benefit.

Man has done much to shift the delicate balance of nature and the planet and he must learn that this can no longer be. Earth has a delicate balance and this balance and harmony must be returned to her on all levels.

Connect with me and the elementals and together we can spread more love and light around planet Earth and the Nature Kingdom so that the healing and cleansing that needs to take place may be achieved in as painless a way as possible. For we do not want to cause pain and misery to those who reside on Earth but when man does not listen Gaia expects action to be taken for the situation that is currently on Earth cannot be allowed to continue.

Man is no more and no less than any other living being on Earth for we are all one and all come from the same source. It is time for man to realise that true power is not in having power over things and making them feel powerless but true power is standing in light and love so that all living beings receive that love and light and are treated with the respect that they deserve.

We want Earth to be a place filled with love, light, joy and peace and to that end we will do what it takes to make man listen and realise that he is not the master of the world, but is an equal part of it and needs to work in love and harmony with the planet and all those who reside on her'

Channelled by Sarah Hunt 1/8/12

Archangel Butyalil

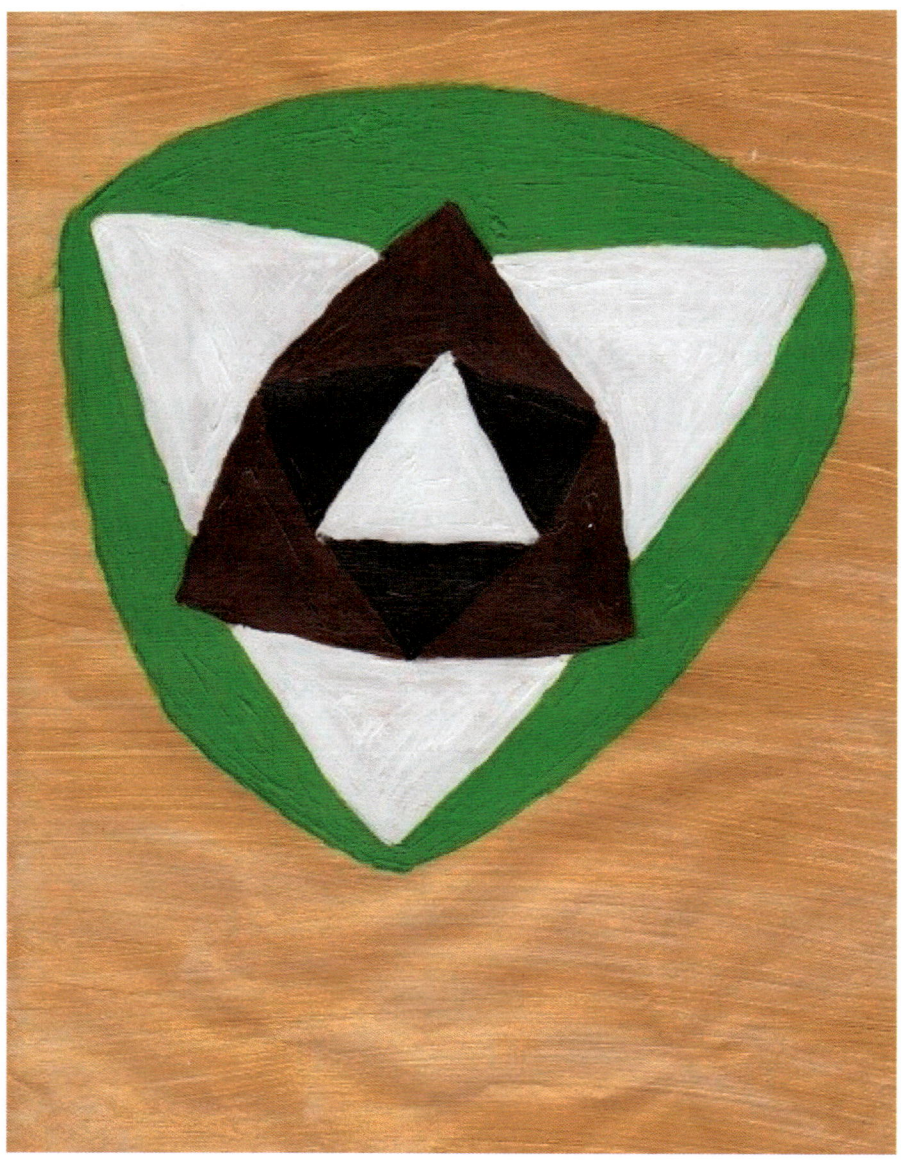

Archangel Butyalil is a Universal Angel who is in charge of the stars and energies around the planet which cause cosmic currents that affect the Earth.

Butyalil is white and carries divine masculine energies. When he comes to planet Earth he steps his energies down through the pyramids in Egypt. Butyalil's role is vast as he not only works with Earth but also works in co-operation with the Archangels of other planets as well as Purlimiek and the Nature Kingdom.

The unicorns, Archangel Metatron and Seraphim Seraphima all actively work with him as well. His twin flame is Archangel Gersisa who works with Archangels Sandolphon and Roquiel to clear mankind's Earth Star chakras so that more light can be brought into Mother Earth. She also ensures that the ley lines are cleansed by using the energy of the full moon to strengthen and align the planetary grid.

I am Butyalil and it is with great love that I am here with you today for there is work to be done to assist Gaia with her ascension process. My work is indeed vast but as you connect with me you can also connect with my twin flame Archangel Gersisa for she too needs your assistance. The energy grids in and around the Earth need to be cleansed so that we can strengthen and realign them, in order to assist the ascension process. More light must be brought into Mother Earth herself and you can assist this process by clearing and cleansing your Earth Star chakra so that more light can be anchored into the Earth through you.

Spend time out in nature connecting with the plants and animals. As you make time to do this you will feel the energies moving through you to assist Mother Earth. Allow us to work through you and with you so that we can strengthen the energy grids of the planet and so that more light may be brought into Earth to assist the cleansing process that must take place. For as we work together we can make this process a smoother one than it otherwise might need to be.

Work on yourself as well, for as you lift your vibration you will be able to carry and indeed anchor more light into the Earth. This is key in the ascension process. Although I work within the universe I am never far away and will work with you to bring balance and harmony to Mother Earth on all levels.

There are many places on your planet that need more light and many situations have been created to achieve this but if darkness or fear creep in then more drastic action will need to take place. We want to work with you for the greater good of all and to show mankind that he is not here to have control over Mother Earth or the energies and resources within and around her, but to work in harmony and love with all who reside on her so that all may benefit and achieve their highest potential.'

Channelled by Sarah Hunt 1/8/12

Archangel Gersisa

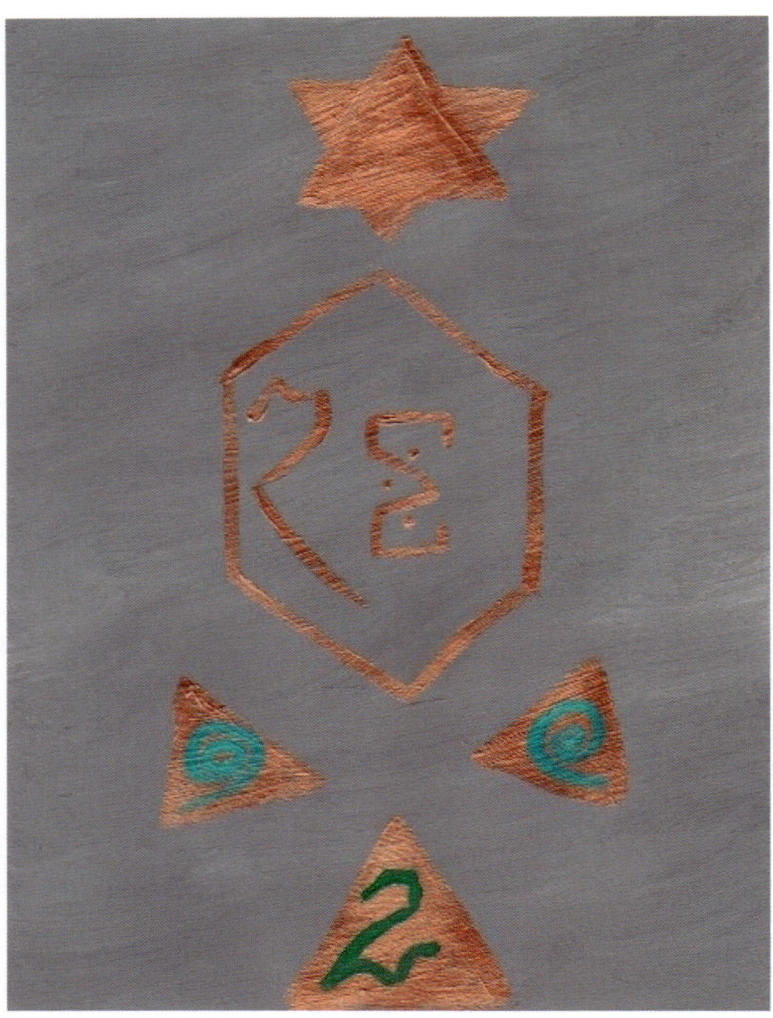

Archangel Gersisa is Archangel Butyalil's twin flame and carries the Divine Feminine energies. She connects with those above the Earth as well as those within it. Her retreat is within Middle (Hollow) Earth which is within the very core of the planet.

She assists Archangels Sandolphon and Roquiel with clearing our Earth Star chakras. She wants us to self-heal as well so that we can hold more light which will enable us to channel more light into the Earth as our Earth Star chakras are cleared.

Within Middle Earth her role is to look after the leylines, helping to keep them cleansed. She also works with the planetary energy grid and works with the energies of the moon to keep the grid strong and aligned. She works closely with the Elemental Master Taia to do this.

'I am Gersisa and it is with great love that I am here with you today. I work with Gaia and am helping her to clear the negativity within the planet. I also work with my Twin Flame Butyalil who works with the cosmic energies. 'As above so below'. As this spiritual law states by working with the energies of the inner planes as well as the outer planes, we in the Angelic and Elemental Realms are able to balance the energy grids. The energies above therefore match the energies below.

There are many new energies coming into the Earth and indeed they are coming from the cosmos but be aware that there are also energies coming from Middle Earth to you as well.

It is important for you to look within and heal yourself for the chaos on the planet is as a result of the chaos that man has within. It is the collective energies that are causing the chaos on the Earth plane so it is important for as many light workers as possible to work to heal themselves, as well as others, so that as a collective you start to create the world of peace and love that so many of you truly desire.

We will and are working with you for this too is our vision, this too is what we wish to create. For when there is peace and love from within then there is oneness. A oneness with yourself as well as with the universe.

Do not be afraid to go into the darkest corners of your soul, for you are a being of love and light and you have the tools to illumine the darkest parts of you, the part that some refer to as your shadow self. Used in the right way with the right intent, the energies of the shadow self can bring great strength but used in the wrong way they can bring destruction.

Open your heart and let divine love in, allow the flow of love from you to the universe and from the universe to you so that you can heal and bring yourself to a place of wholeness, peace and love.

As you do this you will attract peace and love around you and find yourself living a far more positive life. The more people that achieve this the quicker we will be able to help Mother Earth to clear the energies of darkness and bring love light and peace to all who reside on her. '

Channelled by Sarah Hunt 15/11/14

I am going to include Gaia in this section as well and whilst she is not classed as an angel, but as a goddess, you can connect with her to gain guidance with how she wishes for you to work with her to assist the ascension process.

Gaia works closely with each of the angels and Elemental Masters that I have included in this book and so has a very important role in the ascension process. She of course knows exactly what needs to be done for Earth to ascend.

Gaia

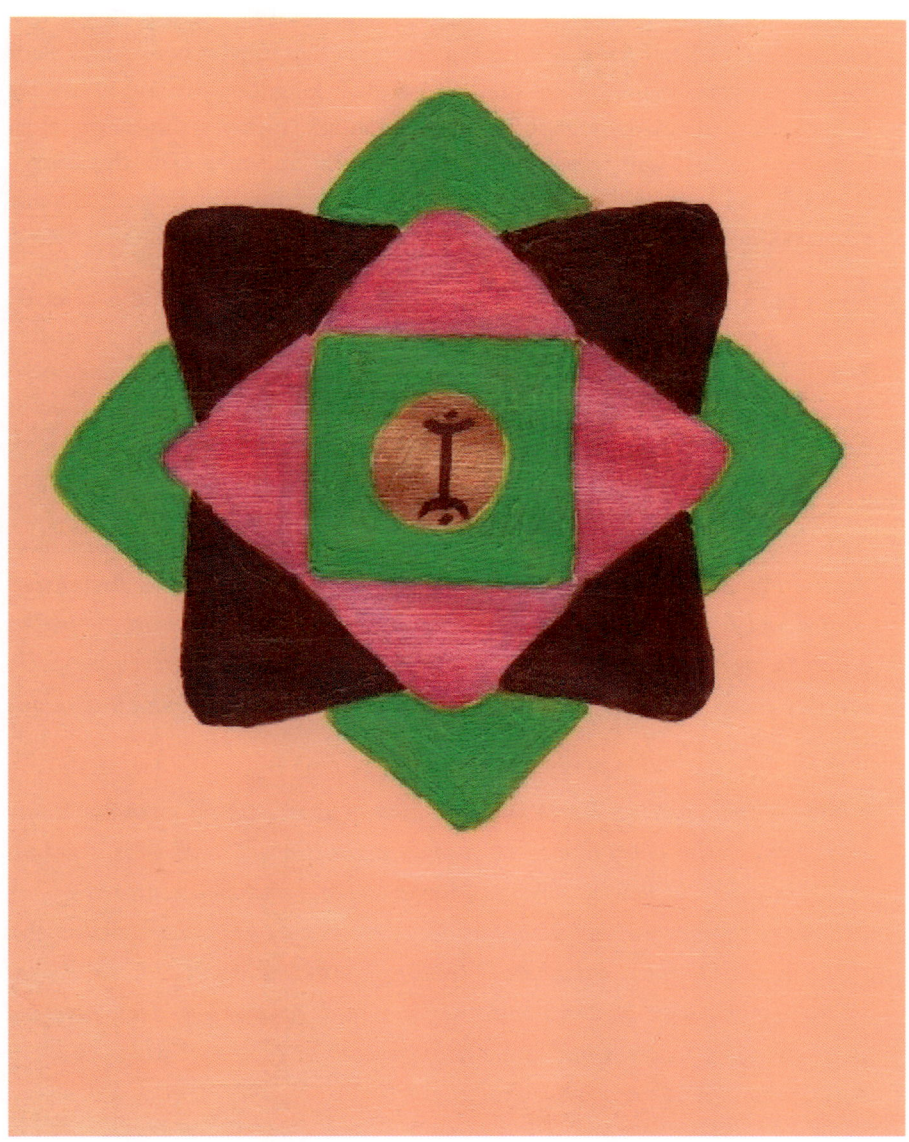

Gaia is the principle energy responsible for the Earth and has decreed (and so it must be) that Earth will ascend.

Gaia is fertility itself for mankind, the creatures that inhabit her and all plant forms. She gives mankind, the animal and plant kingdom, life and nourishes and nurtures them throughout life. In death she receives the empty shell back into herself and transforms it to new life. She maintains the eternal rhythmic balance so that all life thrives. She protects that balance fiercely when necessary.

Some see Gaia as a goddess and indeed in some mythology she is referred to as a goddess but for me she is so much more. She is a vast expansive energy filled with love who wants to move Earth into a new dimension so that peace and harmony reign once more. She will use tough love if necessary so that mankind will listen and once more show respect and love to Gaia, the planet and all who reside on her.

'It is with great love that I am here with you today for there is much work to be done. I have decreed that Earth will ascend and indeed that process has already started and is much further on than many people realise. Not enough people are seeing the signs or listening to their intuition about the ascension process for if they did they would realise that it has moved much further and more quickly than was originally intended.

There are many souls on Earth who have come to assist with the ascension process and there are also many who think that ascension is about man. This is not the case. Humans still have so much to learn about love and the importance of love and many humans will not ascend for they have not yet grasped the lessons that they have come to learn, but whatever happens Earth will ascend as it was decreed by me that this must happen. Earth has been ready to ascend for some time and so the process was accelerated by her willingness to let go of that which no longer serves her so that she could truly heal.

It has become very apparent to those of us beyond the veil that the most important thing is love, divine love as this is unconditional love. Divine love heals everything and so I ask you to help Mother Earth by anchoring divine love into her so that she may be cleansed and healed which in turn will allow her to ascend further. Some people think that the Earth will ascend to the fifth dimension and indeed she has reached that level but is ascending further. Ascension is a continual process for all of us and will continue until we have learnt all our lessons from all parts of the universe and will continue until we are ready to return to Source.

It is also important to show Mother Earth respect and thanks. Man has spent too much time disrespecting Mother Earth and abusing her resources. He has allowed ego to get in the way and as a result of this has tried to disempower the Earth instead of working with her in love and harmony. Man has allowed greed and gluttony to take over instead of only using the resources offered by the Earth that he really needs.

He has forgotten the importance of thanking Mother Earth for all the resources that she offers to man to help him to live on her. He takes for granted the fact that Mother Earth provides him with everything he needs to reside on her, his food and shelter, his clothes. He does not take the time to see the beauty in the simple things that surround him but looks for more and more materialistic wealth. Man needs to go within and look at himself for when he does this and connects with who he truly is he will start to see the beauty within and then he will see the beauty of the world that surrounds him.

When was the last time that you stopped to admire the sunset or watch a bird as it hovers on a thermal in the air? When was the last time that you thanked Mother Earth for the beauty around you, for the food and water and the shelter that she provides you with? When did you last look at the simple things in life and realise that they are what is important? When did you last realise how much the Earth supports you? When did you last realise how much Mother Earth loves you?

We are truly blessed to be working with Mother Earth whether incarnate or beyond the veil for she has much to teach us all. It is time for everyone to realise this and to treat her with the love and respect that she deserves and to move towards living in peace and harmony with her so that we can all grow and ascend together.'

Channelled from Gaia 4/1/13 by Sarah Hunt

You can work with these Angels and Gaia as a group or individually. Just simply invoking them by calling their name with love and gratitude will bring them to you. You may also find that they appear in situations where they are able to help you as you may have requested their assistance on a deeper level. They will guide you as to how they wish to work with you, which may be through self-healing, healing animals, healing the world or working with them when you are healing others (for those of you who are healers) or working with them when you are out in nature. The important thing is to trust that they will guide you as to how they want you to work with them and then allow them to work with you and through you in whatever way is right for you.

THE ELEMENTAL MASTERS

Elementals are made up of at least one of the elements, i.e. earth, wind, water or fire. Some of them contain more than one element and others may be any of the different elements.

The Elemental Masters that I have been guided to work with for this book are Dom, The Elemental Master of air, Thor, the Elemental Master of fire, Neptune the Elemental Master of water, Merlin the Elemental Master of earth (here I am talking about the element earth not planet earth!) and Taia the Elemental Master of Middle Earth. There are, I am sure, many other Elemental Masters who each have an important role' but these are the ones I have been working with for a while, who have given me healing images, messages and meditations to bring to you. Taia is a new Elemental Master who connected with me recently. I understand I am to introduce you to Taia in this book and that there will be more to bring to you in a later book, yet to be written.

Here is a message that I channelled from Archangel Purlimiek, Lady Gaia, Dom, Neptune, Thor and Merlin in 2013

There are going to be many large energetic shifts in order for Mother Earth to heal. These too will be lessons for man so that he realises that he can no longer continue to abuse Mother Earth and her resources and that he must learn to work in harmony with her and all who reside on her. It is time for man to realise that he is not superior to Mother Earth or to any other living being who resides on Earth, but that he is in fact equal to each and every other living being whether they reside on Earth in a physical form or whether they work from beyond the veil.

The energy system of Mother Earth needs to be restored and the land and waters need to be cleansed. We can all work together to achieve this by bringing in love to Mother Earth and by treating every living being with love, including yourselves. It is important to learn to love yourself and accept yourself for who you are. As you learn to love yourself and accept yourself you will learn the importance of accepting all living beings for who they are too.

Only then will you truly see the beauty of the world around you for there is beauty within everything and everyone if you are willing to see it. There is love within everything and everyone if you are willing to accept it. When we learn to love ourselves we are then able to truly love others, for it is love which is important. It is love that surrounds us at every part of our journey whether on Earth or in other parts of the universe. It is love which is eternal, it is love which connects us all, but for this to happen we all need to learn to give and receive love, for there has to be a balance in the giving and receiving of love. When we are able to do this we are able to see that love has no boundaries but is infinite and limitless and can help to change you and the world around you.

When we find the love that is within each of us we are able to project love and the world around us becomes more loving and peaceful. So this is our message to you learn to love yourselves so that you may love others. Learn to receive love as well as to give it and recognise that the only thing that is real is love, the only thing that is important is love the one thing that can heal everything is love. When we focus on love we can bring about a truly peaceful and happy world. We ask you to work with us to heal the world and those who reside on her with love.
We love and honour you and thank you for working with us.'

Channelled by Sarah Hunt 4/1/13

Here is a message from these beautiful beings brought to me today whilst writing this book.

'It is with great love that we are here with you today for there is much to be done. Mother Earth is indeed ascending and will continue to do so for some time. This process was started some time ago and is indeed progressing far better than any of us anticipated.

Gaia has decreed that Earth must ascend and so it must and will be.
Many on Earth at the present moment are here to assist with the ascension process and to help Mother Earth with her healing. Many who are here for that purpose have not yet awoken but this will not hinder things for the process has already begun and is far more advanced than we expected it to be.

Mother Earth needs love and light to be sent to her and channelled into her so that we in the world of spirit can anchor the energies into her. This will enable the transmutation of many negative energies that are deep within her energies to be dissolved and transmuted so that her vibration may lifted yet further. As her vibration lifts, as with any other being of light, she will be able to hold and radiate more light.

There are many energetic shifts taking place currently and many dramas being played out. Many on Earth do not understand what is happening but it is old energy being cleared. As with any form of healing, in order to become whole once again things appear to get worse before they can get better. This is just part of the cleansing process.

Many of you have assisted with this process in other parts of the universe and will remember the shifts that need to take place for progress to be made.
Each and every one of you must continue to heal yourselves, for if you want to attain peace on Earth then you must find peace within yourself. If you want to be loved and be surrounded by love then you must learn to love yourself and surround yourself with love. Self-healing is therefore key for each and every one of you if you are to attain the peace and love that your heart desires.

We will also work with you and guide you with assisting Mother Earth with her healing, all you need to do is ask. As we work together as one we create a greater healing force than each of us as individuals is able to. Together we will make Earth a place filled with love. Together we will ascend into a new dimension and a new more spiritual way of being. Together we will bring peace to all on Earth. For we are all one and we are all love.

Channelled from the Nature Angels and Elemental Masters by Sarah Hunt 5/11/14

The Elemental Masters just like the angels have to work with the spiritual laws and can only help us if we ask them to. This is the **Law of Request**. They too, like the angels, like to be appreciated and thanked so always ensure that you thank them when you have finished working with them or when you see something of beauty in the world. This is the **Law of Gratitude.**

In the recent message they have stated that Lady Gaia has decreed that Earth must ascend. This is the **Law of Decree.** As Gaia has decreed that Earth will ascend then the universe will align itself to ensure that this will happen.

Understanding the Laws of the Universe can help you to understand how to work with those that are in spirit ready and waiting to work with you. When we work with the spiritual laws we step into the flow of our lives and empower those in spirit whether angels, elementals, Ascended Masters or any other being of light to work with us for the highest good of all.

Dom, Elemental Master of Air

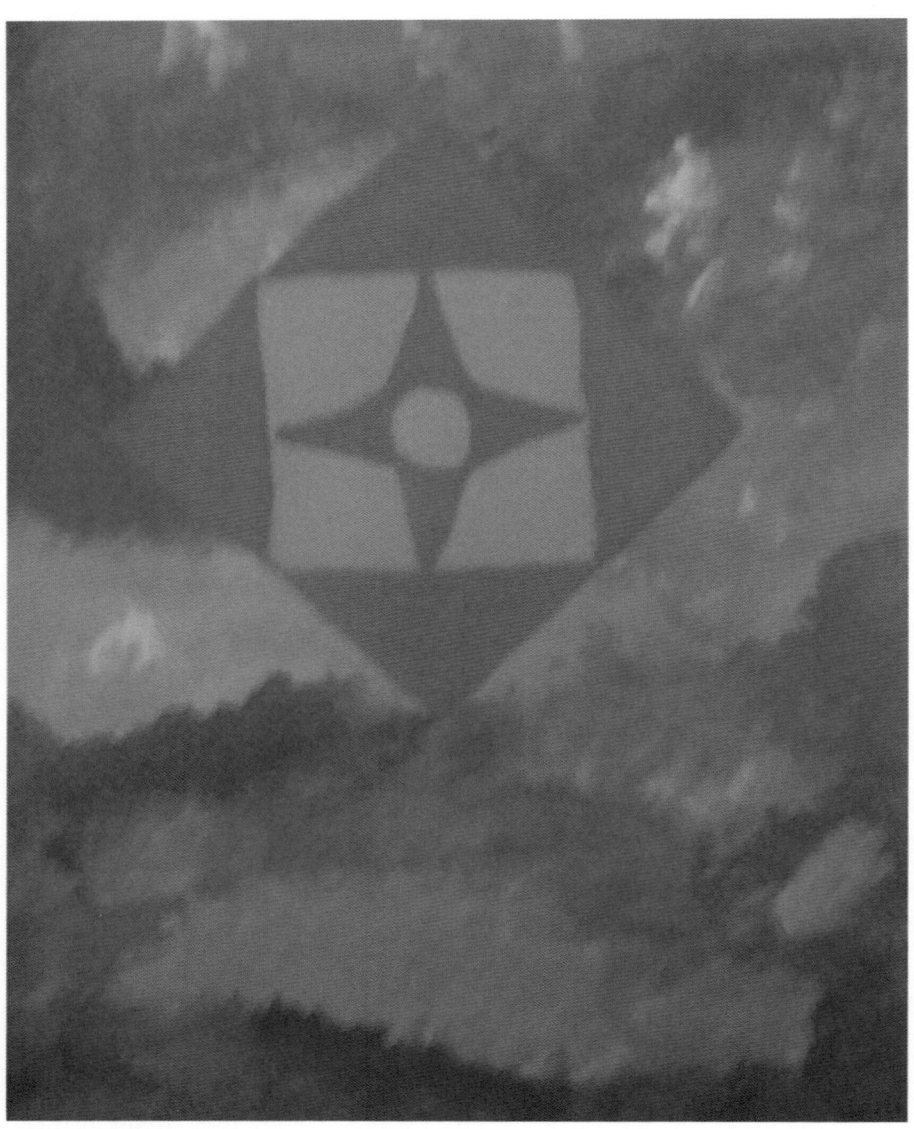

Dom is the Elemental Master of Air and has a quiet yet vast presence. He manages the sylphs who affect the winds. If you take the time to stand in the wind and feel it you will notice each wind is and feels different.

The sylphs help to clear the negativity in the air by affecting the winds. They also move oxygen, carbon dioxide and carbon monoxide around the planet so that the air is balanced. Trees and plants will convert carbon dioxide to oxygen but man has cleared a lot of the vegetation and trees and so they are not as able to contribute to rebalancing the oxygen levels as they used to be, so it needs to be done in other ways. This is where Dom and the sylphs come in as they are able to move the oxygen and carbon dioxide/monoxide so that the balance within the air is redressed. Dom works closely with Lady Gaia to assist the Earth by ensuring the air is balanced.

When it is particularly stormy and the winds are high there is a need for a large amount of healing to take place through the winds. Send out love and light to Dom and the sylphs and you will be sure to assist the healing process and help to reduce the strength of the winds needed for the cleansing process.

'I am Dom and it is with great love that I am with you today for there is a great need for the air on this planet to be balanced and cleansed of all negativity. Mankind has not understood the importance of the balance of the air and has changed the landscapes by removing plants and cutting down trees. This part of nature not only helps to protect the Earth with its physical presence but by the biological sequences which take part within them so that the balance of oxygen and carbon dioxide is correct.

The sylphs are the elementals of the air and work with me with the winds and Lady Gaia to ensure that balance is maintained and that negativity is transmuted to love. Take the time to stand in the wind and truly feel it for it will give you a greater sense of Mother Earth and the work that needs to be done to assist her healing and her ascension. Know that it is love that is needed to heal her and all who reside on her and open your heart centre to assist with this process, sending love to Mother Earth to assist this process.

Feel the wind cleanse the Earth and you, for when you are out in the wind it will help you to clear your own energy system of any negativity that has become stuck within it. There is still a lot of work to be done for man has created a lot of imbalance and negativity around and within the Earth which needs to be rebalanced and cleansed. Know that when it is windy you can help us to cleanse the Earth and bring calm by opening your heart chakra and sending love out into and around the Earth, for love heals everything and will expediate the healing process that has been started.'

Channelled by Sarah Hunt 7/1/13

There are other elemental beings who are Air Elementals and work under the guidance of Dom. These include; esaks, elves and fairies.

The Air Elementals

The air elementals true inner nature is related to human will. Their consciousness lives in the airy element of the ether and the term 'will-o'-the-wisp' gives an indication of the true nature of the air spirits.

Sylphs

Sylphs are air spirits that work with flowers and plants like the fairies. They clear the pollution around plants to help to keep them healthy. They love to fly in the wind. You can also call in the sylphs to help to cleanse your aura and clear the 'cobwebs' from your mind. They are looked after by Dom who is the Elemental Master of the Air. When it is really windy Dom will be working with the sylphs to cleanse the air and the Earth. You can ask them to do their cleansing in a more gentle way so that the wind drops.

Sylphs, under the guidance of Dom will also help to redress the balance of oxygen and carbon dioxide. This has become a task that they do more often now due to the way that the habitat has changed leaving us with fewer plants and trees to convert carbon dioxide to oxygen. So where there are pockets of either too much oxygen or too much carbon dioxide or too many of any of the other elements that make up the air, the sylphs will help to move the air around to change the balance of those elements.

The balance of air is important as all living beings need air in some form to be able to breathe and live. When it is very windy connect with the Sylphs and ask them to allow you to work with them. Send them unconditional love and send love out into the air so that it dissolves any negativity that is floating around in it.

The sylphs also bring light through the element of air in order to assist the natural processes of the earth. Sylphs are felt to be highly sensitive to the sun and sensitive to the alignment of the planets and so influenced by both the sun and the planets. They are said to bring universal will, love and the wisdom of the cosmos into the element of air.

Due to pollution there is a reduction not just in oxygen in the air but also of the amount of pure sunlight that is able to get through to the planet which of course adds to the workload of the sylphs.

The sylphs are in a constant state of movement and are involved in bringing information in from the cosmos into the etheric levels of the plant life as well as the air.

We can help the sylphs by connecting with them and working from our hearts sending pure love and healing out into the air to assist them with their work.

Esaks

Esaks have recently been invited to assist with cleansing the planet and come from a different universe. Their task is to vacuum up negative energy so that the new higher frequencies can come in. We can work with them as well by asking to work with them and sending out love to any areas that they are cleansing.

Elves

Elves live in the element air, and are like light in the atmosphere. They are sensitive to the movement of the atmosphere and have a sleepy consciousness. Their task is to transfer light to the plants. The stream of air caused by a flying bird creates a sound they can hear. Elves are more connected to the expansion of life in their area whilst Sylphs are more connected to movement in space.

Fairies

Fairies are of the element air and tend flowers. They are delightful, pure, innocent, playful creatures who love to play and tease, but are never malicious. They are a very friendly group of elementals who love to be spoken to and asked to help. Fairies are very powerful manifestors and know that through the processes of firm belief and clear visualisation they can attract what they want into their lives. The fairies on Earth are ready to work with humans with a pure heart to teach us about their powerful manifestation skills and using the moon cycles to harness the available energy here on Earth.

They are also keen to help us heal our hearts and to find love in everything and every situation. They find it painful to watch humans' behaviour towards one and other and towards animals and nature. Fairies live in big collective groups, and like to socialise, party and have fun together. They always see the love in every situation however they do get annoyed when we show no respect for planet Earth, which is why they have a mischievous reputation.

You can easily connect with the Fairy Realm by sitting amongst flowers and plants and quietening your mind. You may wish to hold a piece of rose quartz or amethyst crystal as the fairies are very attracted to them. Fairies connect with us through our clairsentience which allows us to receive messages through feelings. So as you connect with the Fairy Realm open your heart and allow them to come to you. Fairies can truly see who we are, so if you have any problems or tendencies you know are not serving you well, you can ask them to help you to heal them. They will transmute any pain or negative beliefs to light and help us to see a better way of being.

I have a very beautiful fairy who works with me especially when I am healing others. Her name is Anya and she is very playful. She showed herself to one of my students at a workshop one day. I asked this student if she was ok because she kept looking at me in a funny way. She told me that she kept seeing something darting backwards and forwards behind me a bit like Tinkerbell in Peter Pan! I realised then that she was seeing my beautiful Fairy Anya.

Meditation

Make yourself comfortable and imagine feel or see a bubble of golden light surrounding you keeping you safe. Take a moment to focus on your breathing, becoming aware of each breath in and each breath out. Feel your body and mind start to relax as you focus on your breathing and allow it to move into a slow and steady rhythm.

Now become aware of Dom the Elemental Master of the air, feel his beautiful light energy surrounding you. As your awareness of Dom heightens you realise that there are many other beings there too, sylphs, esaks, elves and fairies are all there waiting to work with you.

Dom asks you to spend some time with the sylphs first of all. No sooner has he told you that this is what he wants than you find yourself whisked away with the sylphs, flying through the air with them. As you do this allow your heart to open and send love and light out from your heart centre so that you are assisting the sylphs as they take you with them and show you how they work. Stay with the sylphs for the next few minutes and allow them to take you wherever they need to go...........

The sylphs take you back to where Dom is and he thanks you for assisting them. He then asks the esaks to take you with them. Continue to keep your heart centre open and send out love and light as you spend the next few moments with the esaks. Watch how they work and ask them what you can do to help them. ....

The esaks take you back to Dom and he now asks you to spend some time with the elves. Whilst they appear to have a sleepy consciousness notice how sensitive to the movement of air they are. Watch how they transfer light to the plants and ask them what you can do to help them........

The elves return you to Dom and now you are asked to spend some time with the fairies. Find yourself moving around the flowers with the fairies and watch how they work with plants and the Earth. Connect with the fairies and ask them to work with you and guide you. Ask them what you can do to help them and ask them to help you. Continue to send both love and light from your heart centre as you work with the fairies.

The fairies take you back to Dom and he gives you an opportunity to ask questions. Ask him anything you want to know so that you can help the Air Elementals to heal the Earth as well as help yourself with your own healing.

Thank Dom and each of the elementals for showing you how they work and bring yourself back to this time and space grounding yourself by imagining roots going out from your feet down into the centre of Mother Earth, wrapping around the amethyst crystal at the centre of the Earth, so that you are completely grounded and connected and then open your eyes when you feel ready.

Neptune, Elemental Master of Water

Neptune is the Elemental Master of the waters and works with the mermaids, mermen, sprites, kyphils and undines to clear the waters and move them. Many people think of the seas when they think of Neptune but it is my understanding that he works with the elementals with any expanses of water so that will include lakes and rivers as well. Part of Neptune's work includes working with Lady Gaia to affect and direct the rain so that water can help to cleanse areas of land.

' I am Neptune and it is with great love that I am here with you today for it is important for you to understand the need for us to work together to clear the waters of the Earth of all the negativity and pollution that has been caused by man. I work with many different water elementals within the expanses of water to assist with cleansing process which is required to assist Mother Earth with her ascension.

Man has created a lot of pollution within the waters of the Earth and does not realise the importance of balance within the waters. He over fishes areas too and appears to be oblivious to the need for balance within the waters to ensure that the food chain is complete. Many creatures are being affected by man's misuse of the fruits of the waters and by his misunderstanding and fear of many of the animal groups which reside within water. Man feels a need to have power over these creatures and has not realised that we are all equal and that we all need to live in harmony with each other. Love, harmony and balance are what are important between all living beings and it is time for man to realise and understand this.

Many of you will question the need for the natural disasters which have happened and certainly when you look from a 3D point of view they seem to be horrific situations, however they are necessary to cleanse the Earth of all the negativity and destruction that man has caused. They are necessary to rebalance the karmic debt between man and Earth. They are also necessary to teach man how to love and be compassionate towards others and to understand the need to work together for the good of all. Man still has many many lessons to learn so that he realises that he is an equal part of life on Earth and needs to live in harmony with all life and with Earth and that he must not abuse the Earth but care for her and ensure that he uses her resources wisely.

There needs to be much more of a balance of giving and receiving between man and Mother Earth and man needs to learn the importance of love and both giving and receiving unconditional love to every living being, for even the smallest creature on the Earth is as important as man and has a contribution to make to the balance of Earth and the lives of all those living beings who reside on her.

I work with Mother Earth and the elementals of water to assist in cleansing the planet through the rains as well as working directly in each expanse of water to cleanse, clear and rebalance it. It is important to fill the planet with love to achieve the cleansing and balance that is required for Mother Earth to continue to ascend. '
    Channelled by Sarah Hunt 7/1/13

The Water Elementals

Mermaids and Mermen

Mermaids and mermen are the guardians of the seas and look after the whales, dolphins, sharks, seals, porpoises, fish and turtles and any other sea dwelling creatures. They are very friendly elementals and you are most likely to find them on rocks out in the sea but they live all over.

Mermaids are trying to get our attention at this time to heal the seas and work in harmony with the ocean sprites whose job it is to energetically purify the water. They will also assist with healing emotional problems and traumas in humans. Mermaid energy is very soothing.

They are particularly concerned about how the oil spillages, chemical spillages, chemical dumping, sewage dumping and missile testing is affecting the delicate balance of our seas. They also have grave concerns about the coral which is being bleached, the overfishing and whale killings. Whales and Dolphins are highly evolved creatures who carry special frequencies on Earth as do sharks. They all work on a very high vibration.

Undines

The undines also live in the oceans and they look after the underwater plants and also the energy ley lines. Their job is to keep the ley lines free so that Mother Earth can send her energy along them. The undines also live in fresh water and look like mermaids except that they have legs instead of tails. They are concerned that the natural world beneath our seas and rivers is in energetic and physical turmoil due to the chemicals from factories and fields as well as the salinity changes in the oceans and the temperature rises that are taking place.

Plants, coral and kelp are dying off and these are needed to help with the energetic purification of our waters. The knock on effect of this is that the natural hunting grounds of the animals and fish that live in the waters are changing. They need our help to redress the balance in the waters of the Earth.

Kyphils

Kyhils like esaks have also come from another universe and their task is to clear the negative energies in the waters of the world.

Meditation

Make yourself comfortable so that you can completely relax and put your protection around you. Take some deep breaths breathing in relaxation, breathing out any tension and allow your body and mind to completely relax.

Now imagine feel or see yourself on the banks of a river and invoke an undine by calling her to you. Imagine feel or see the undine presenting herself to you at the water's edge. Tell her that you have come to assist her with cleansing the waters in front of you.

The undine tells you to get into the water and swim with her as together you can cleanse this water. Know that you are perfectly safe and will be able to breathe under the water. Find yourself in the water swimming with the undine. Be aware of the water around you, is it clear, muddy, silted, dirty or polluted.

As you breathe in draw in a beautiful pink light from the universe which is filled with love and as you breathe out see yourself breathing this beautiful pink light into the water. Watch as the energies of the water are transmuted and cleansed. See the water becoming clear once more. Keep swimming around the water with the Undine breathing in the pink light filled with love and breathing it out into the water.

If you come across any animals that live in the water who look as if they are ill, heal them by breathing this beautiful pink light around them so that you purify their energy with the loving energy you are channelling from the universe. Be open to any messages that these creatures may wish to impart to you in the form of pictures, words or feelings which may help you to understand how else you can help to heal the waters of the Earth.

As you swim around become aware of the pattern of the ley lines and notice any which seem to be blocked. Breathe the cleansing pink light into the ley line to clear it and watch as the unconditional love within the pink light dissolves any blockages within the ley lines.

As you swim along the river with the undine, you explain to her that you also want to assist with healing the oceans. The undine explains that the mermaids and mermen will be glad of your assistance and tells you that she will take you along the river until it reaches the ocean. As you swim along the river with the undine you continue to breathe in the pink light filled with love form the universe and breathe it out into the water surrounding you.

As you reach the mouth of the river where it meets the ocean the undine tells you that she is going to take you to meet a mermaid.

You swim a bit further with the undine and then find yourself surrounded by mermaids and mermen. They are pleased to see you and want to work with you to help the polluted waters.

The undine thanks you for your help in the river and waves good bye to you. You thank the undine and then ask the mermaids and mermen how you can help them to cleanse the oceans.

Listen to what they say to you. Allow them to show you what you can do to help them with this cleansing process and spend some time working with them with this.

Be aware of the energies of the waters as you start to work with the mermaids and mermen. Notice how they appear to you and notice how they change as you work together.

The mermaids and mermen are happy with the work that you have done together and one of them tells you that he/she will take you back to the mouth of the river to meet with the undine again.

You swim with the mermaid until once again you connect with the undine. The mermaid thanks you for helping them and you thank her for the opportunity. The undine tells you to come with her and she takes you back to the part of the river where you originally started. You thank the undine for bringing you back safely and you swim back up to the surface of the water.

You climb back onto the bank of the river and find that you are immediately dry as you stand on the river bank in the sun thinking about the wonderful experiences you have just had.

Now bring yourself back to this time and space grounding yourself before opening your eyes.

Merlin Elemental Master of Earth

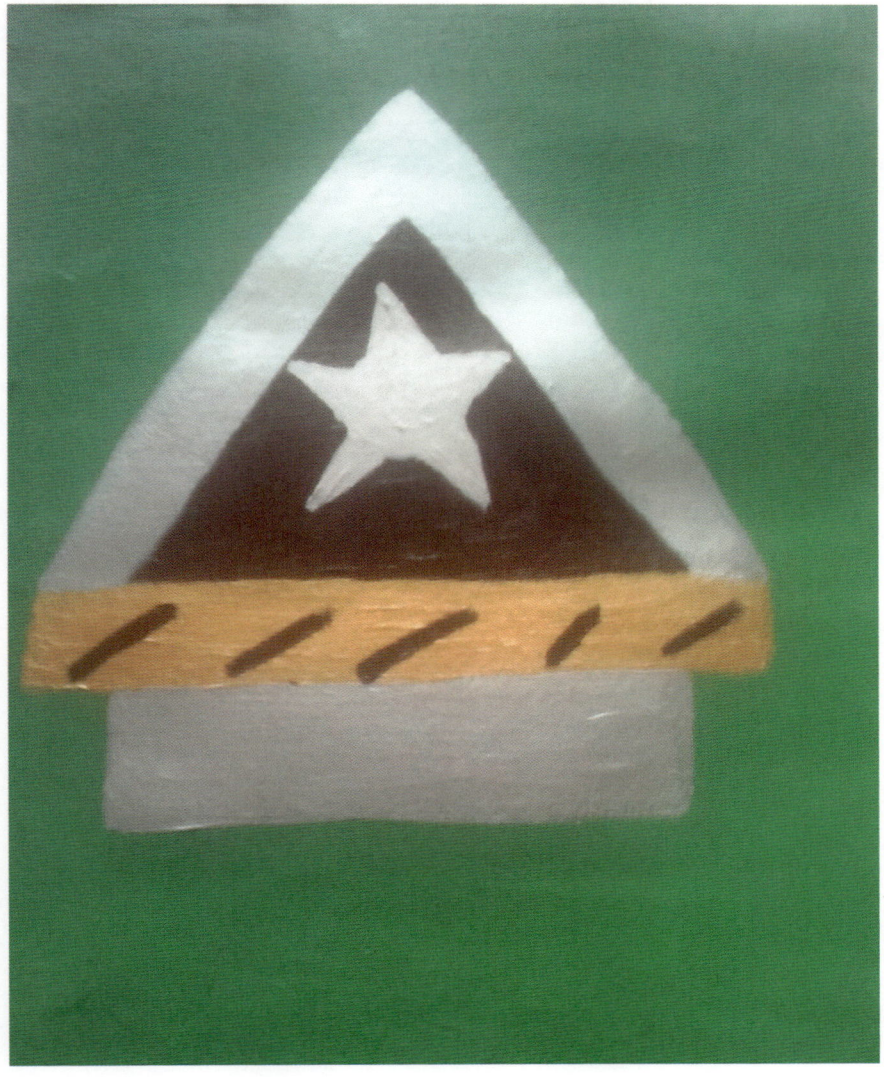

Merlin is an interesting character who has been surrounded by a lot of myth over centuries. He is probably best known as a wizard with great powers who was supposed to have protected King Arthur.

From the connections that I have now made with Merlin it is my belief that the stories around King Arthur are all myth and King Arthur didn't actually ever exist. Merlin however I feel was a very gifted healer who worked closely with some important people in Avalon. He may have been seen as magical because of the wonderful gifts that he had. He has an amazing connection with Mother Earth and not only worked with healing energies but also with herbs and plants to assist people's healing.

Merlin may be seen as everything, i.e. he is the Earth, humanity and underlies all life on Earth. He is one of the custodians of Earth as well as an advisor and a guardian of Earth and so has a deep connection with the element earth as well as our beloved planet.

Since connecting with Merlin I have become aware that he is the Elemental Master who works with the earth elementals such as pixies, elves and gnomes. I also feel that he has a very close connection with dragons too and dragons may be made up of any of the four elements.
Merlin works with Gaia with earthquakes, Tsunamis and volcanic eruptions to assist with the cleansing process.

It is with great love that I am with you today and I am very aware that there are many myths surrounding my very existence. However what is important is the now and working together to assist Mother Earth with her healing and her ascension. I am the Elemental Master of the Earth and work with those spirits who are connected with the Earth such as fairies, pixies and elves. We work closely with Lady Gaia to assist Mother Earth with her healing and her ascension process. It is important that you connect with these beings for they are the guardians of the Earth and will teach you how to love and care for the Earth and work in harmony with her.

It is important for man to respect Mother Earth and to use her resources wisely and to give back to Earth as well as take from her. The elementals will assist you with understanding the need for this to happen as well as help you to understand the healing that needs to take place within the Earth herself as a result of the way she has been treated by man. It is important for us to all work together from the heart with love to assist the Earth at this time.

Remember too the importance of healing yourself and of receiving as well as giving love. It is divine love which will heal everything both for man and for Earth and we are all in a truly interesting time as we work together to assist the ascension of this beautiful planet.'

Channelled by Sarah Hunt 10/1/13

Earth Elementals

Pixies — animals

Pixies help to maintain the quality of the soil and rove in bands. They remind us of the importance of nurturing and blessing the ground. They also remind us that connecting with the Earth assists us with grounding and allowing our true light to shine. Pixies never stay in one place for long as they are trouble shooters assisting with the quality of the soil and helping to prevent soil erosion. They are also the guardians of animals and their role to animals is rather like the role of our guardian angel, i.e. to keep the animal safe and make sure it doesn't pass until it is its time to go. Pixies are very keen on stressing how important it is for humans to be kind and loving to all animals and are passionate about animal welfare and protection. Pixies will work with you to help heal animals and to encourage you in the right direction with regard to your soul's divine path. The Pixies are very friendly elementals and like to work with humans who love animals. Pixies are also passionate about the way wild animals are treated so if you have rats or mice around ask the pixies to help you to send them to a more suitable environment.

Gnomes

Gnomes too are earth elements and look after metals, ores, minerals and crystals. They also look after tree roots. The majority of gnomes live in the Earth but there are some who live in the forests and take care of the forests on an earth element level. They are said to be about 2 to 3 feet in size and look knotty and gnarled. They can appear quite gruff and don't trust humans very easily. Gnomes are said to have a very clever consciousness and so understand what they hear and see. Their sense and intellect are very strong and they receive cosmic influences and ideas.

So plants receive energies from the universe and these energies then sink into the soil where they are collected by the gnomes and the information from the universe is then passed onto the Earth and all the minerals within her.

Gnomes don't have to think things over like we do. Their knowledge is immediate because they have a universal intellect (i.e. they are completely one with the universe) and they receive this knowledge through their senses. They see humans as incomplete and dumb as we don't have this ability!

Kobolds

Kobolds are smaller than gnomes, and much finer. They are very friendly playful beings and like to help whilst still remaining cautious.

Mountain Devas

Mountain devas are more developed earth devas and work with a whole mountain or mountain ranges.

Tree Spirits

Tree spirits are the consciousness of trees and are also earth elementals. They connect with each other and send messages to each other across the planet.

I am a 'tree lover and hugger'! and love to connect with the tree spirits. They can and will connect with us when we are working with the energies of trees. They are an important part of the Nature Kingdom as they help to look after the trees and they are keen to work with those of us who are passionate about helping Mother Earth and the tree kingdom.

Meditation

Ensure that you are comfortable and surround yourself in the protection which resonates most with you. Take your focus to your breathing and become aware of each breath in and each breath out. Allow your breathing to go into a natural rhythm as you allow your body and mind to relax.

Find yourself out in the countryside walking along a beautiful lane with wild flowers in the hedgerows. It is a beautiful sunny day and there is a warm breeze blowing across your face.

As you walk down the lane you notice a great big oak tree and feel as if it is calling you. It is in the middle of a meadow of long grass which has wild flowers growing in amongst the grass.

You open the gate to the meadow and walk through it closing the gate behind you as you make your way. As you approach the beautiful oak tree you hear the voice of the tree spirit telling you to sit at the foot of the tree and lean against it.

The tree spirit then asks you to allow it to help you clear any negativity in your energy system. You become aware of the negativity leaving your body through your root chakra and moving down into the Earth. The tree spirit explains that the Earth is transmuting the energy and that it will come back to you as positive energy in the form of love.

You become aware of a loving energy entering your energy system through your root chakra and moving up through each chakra and then out into your whole energy system. As this happens you become aware of your heart chakra opening as you send love to the tree spirit and the Earth so that there is a flow of loving energies between you.

You are aware of the healing effect that this is having on the tree, the Earth and yourself.

As the energies continue to flow you connect with both the tree spirit and Gaia and ask them how you can help them with the healing of Mother Earth.

Listen to what they tell you and work with them whilst the energies of Divine love are flowing between you all.

The tree spirit and Gaia thank you for your assistance and you thank them for healing you. You feel the flow of energy stop but as you look around you notice how much brighter everything appears. You are aware that you have lifted your vibration.

You thank the beautiful oak tree and Mother Earth as well and make your way back over the meadow to the gate, walking back through it, closing it carefully behind you. You then make your way back along the country lane in the direction that you came from.

Now start to bring your attention back to your body and this time and space and ground yourself before opening your eyes.

Thor Elemental Master of Fire

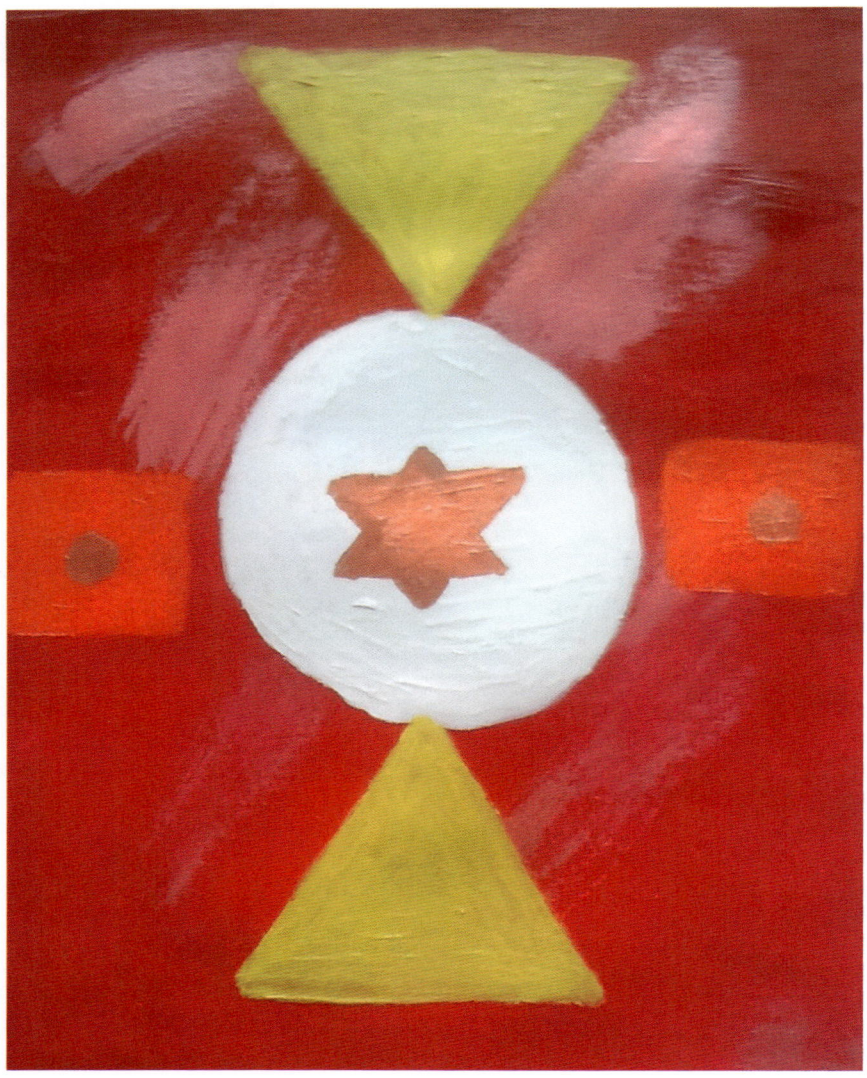

Thor is the Elemental Master of fire and is said to be a Norse (Viking) God who was thought to be the God of Thunder. He was usually portrayed as a large powerful man with a red beard and eyes like lightening. He was popularly thought to be the protector of gods and humans against forces of evil.

Thor as the Elemental Master of Fire, works with forest fires and volcanic eruptions. Like the other Elemental Masters he works closely with the elementals and Mother Earth to bring about the cleansing and clearing that is needed through the different processes.

'I am Thor and I am the Elemental Master for the element fire. Fire is often seen as very destructive by many and certainly when it gets out of control it is a very destructive element. It is however very cleansing and can purify an area which has been filled with negativity.

Fire too can represent the centre of somewhere, the heart of it so to speak. My work is to assist the cleansing of the planet through working with the element of fire. The salamanders work with me and Mother Earth in order to achieve this where this level of cleansing is required.

When a fire is raging send love into its midst so that the area will heal more quickly. Love will help to dissolve the negativity more quickly and so allow the fire to subside more quickly. Together we can heal this planet in a more peaceful way through love and respect being given to Mother Earth herself and all living beings on the planet.'

Channelled by Sarah Hunt 10/1/13

The Fire Elementals

Salamanders

The salamanders work with the fire element and their work is crucial to our existence and the existence of all living things. They infuse the molecules of all matter with the energies necessary to sustain life on Earth and without this spark of life matter would decay, corrode and disintegrate.

Fire is the first step in every process as it provides the initial spark for all life, from the spark of conception of a baby to the spark of inspiration for an idea. Every process begins with the element fire.

Salamanders also control the spiritual-material oscillation of light within the nucleus of every atom and are agents for transferring the fires of the subtle world for mankind's daily use. I.e. electricity, firelight, etc.

They are also responsible for absorbing and transmuting huge masses of negativity over the large cities on Earth and without them, crime and darkness would be much more rampant.

These nature spirits are said to be the biggest, most powerful of the elementals and are also said to be tall, majestic beings appearing as if they are pulsating rainbow fire.

Salamanders can get out of control when they react to human emotions so when there are forest fires raging we can work with them to ask them and help them to calm things down. Sending love and light out to a forest fire will help to dampen it as it will speed up the healing process.

Meditation

Ensure that you are comfortable and put your protection around you. Take some deep breaths and allow your breathing to help you to relax your body and mind. Feel yourself becoming more and more relaxed as your breathing goes into a more relaxed natural rhythm.

Become aware of being out in nature somewhere. You can choose the place that you are in. Look around you and take in all the beautiful sights and sounds of the natural world.

Feel the energies of that beautiful place that you have found. As you look around you notice a tree stump and decide to go and sit on it so that you can connect with that place on a deeper level. Feel yourself becoming one with the beautiful place that you are in.

As you do this you become aware of Thor standing in front of you surrounded by salamanders. Ask Thor how you can help with healing Mother Earth and listen to what he has to say to you.

Spend some time connecting to Thor and listening to what he has to tell you.

Thank Thor for his guidance and then start to become aware of your body once again and bring yourself back to this time and space, grounding yourself before opening your eyes.

Other Elemental Beings

Dragons

Dragons are creatures of all the elements, so they may be earth, air, fire or water. They are beings which have great strength, wisdom and courage. They also offer protection and once you have made a connection with a dragon the bond between you will never break and they will return to you whenever they are needed. They represent the power and transformational energies of the Elemental Kingdom. If you feel drawn to work with dragons then you have a past life connection with them.

It is however very important to offer dragons the utmost respect and usually they will approach you first. They will help you to unlock a lot of spiritual knowledge if you are to work with them providing that you treat them with love and respect.

Unicorns

Unicorns are etheric beings, horses which have fully ascended and belong to the Angelic Realms. The unicorns were present in Atlantis where everyone could connect with them but as the vibration of Atlantis lowered they had to withdraw as they couldn't bring their energy down low enough to be able to continue to connect.

The unicorns have now reappeared in response to prayers for assistance for mankind to ascend. They have been able to reappear as enough people have raised their consciousness for them to be able to come close to the Earth once again.

Unicorns purify us as they remind us of who we truly are. They want to work with those of us who work from the heart and aspire to help others and make the world a better place.

They will hold your vision and give you courage and faith when dealing with challenges that are presented to you. They will give you strength and dignity so that you can fight for what you believe to be right. They encourage you to hold onto your aspirations, visions and ambitions which are for the highest good of all as they have the long term growth of your soul, your community and the world in mind.

Unicorns are seen as white horses with a 'horn' which is actually a spiral of light from their brow chakra. This horn of light pours out divine light and wherever this light is directed healing will take place. They heal not only on a physical and emotional level but on a soul level as well. They are able to dissolve some of the deepest wounds of the soul which may have been carried for many lives. When you are ready the unicorns will help you to clear your karmic debt.

Unicorns reconnect people with their spirit and will align you to the higher realms. If you meet a unicorn in meditation or sleep then your soul is reconnecting with the unicorn energy so that great changes can take place. They will also inspire you behind the scenes.

I connected with my unicorn about three years ago. He is a beautiful being of light called Malchion who often comes to assist me with healings. I recently connected with another unicorn who likes to work with me sometimes and his name is Arjanon.

Unicorns, like angels are androgynous but are often seen as having a feminine energy as the qualities of compassion, wisdom and love are powerful feminine qualities. Unicorns are connected to Source and like angels do not have free will so they will never suggest anything unless it is for the highest good of all and they will never contravene the will of your soul.

Unicorns like angels will leave little white feathers as a sign that they have been with you and are looking out for you. They may also draw your attention to them by bringing your attention to a picture of them or an ornament or a book for example. They also love white flowers.

Unicorns may also have a golden horn and this depicts the great wisdom of a more highly evolved unicorn. It is said that unicorns will grant wishes. In fact what they do is open doors to assist you when you ask from the heart for assistance. They, like the Angelic Realm work with the spiritual laws and cannot help you unless you ask.

There is no limit to the healing that we can do to help Mother Earth. If we connect in with the different elementals during meditation they will guide us with what needs to be done at that particular moment in time. When healing the Earth I like to work with divine (unconditional) love as love heals everything and will bring about the correct balance of energies within the Earth. The Earth also needs light to be anchored into her to assist her with ascension. You can ask the Nature Angels or Elemental Masters to anchor the light into the Earth as you channel it through you into her. Work with your intuition and the guidance of the Nature Angels and Elemental Masters whenever you want to assist Earth with her healing. Remember too that healing yourself is just as important and all these beings of light will assist you with your own healing too.

We each have different elemental guides that will work with us and if we connect with them regularly they will guide and assist us with the healing that needs to take place either on ourselves or with Mother Earth. It is my understanding that we each have one main elemental guide and the others will work alongside this one.

Meditation

Make yourself comfortable so that you can completely relax and put your protection around you. Take some deep breaths breathing in relaxation, breathing out any tension and allow your body and mind to completely relax.

Now imagine feel or see yourself out in a beautiful meadow. The sun is shining and there is a warm breeze on your face. The grass is long around your legs and there are wild flowers growing in amongst the grass.

As you walk across the meadow towards a beautiful Horse Chestnut tree you find yourself wondering whether you have any guides that are elementals who will be able to help you to connect more with the Earth.

As you walk you suddenly become aware of a presence beside you; this is your main elemental guide. Your main elemental guide connects with you and shows you what they are (it may be a sylph, a salamander, a dragon, a fairy or any other elemental). Your elemental guide asks you to come and sit with him under the tree so that you can chat.

Take some time to chat with your main elemental guide to find out more about them. Ask any questions that you feel you need answering to help you to assist with connecting more closely with Mother Earth and healing her.

Your elemental guide then asks you to work with him to help with healing Mother Earth. Listen to what he asks you to do and work with him for the next few minutes. Allow yourself to work from the heart with the intention that the healing that takes place is for the highest good of all.

Now thank your elemental guide for connecting with you and working with you.

Say your good byes and walk back across the meadow to where you started from.

Now bring yourself back to this time and space, grounding yourself before opening your eyes.

Taia Elemental Master of Middle (Hollow) Earth

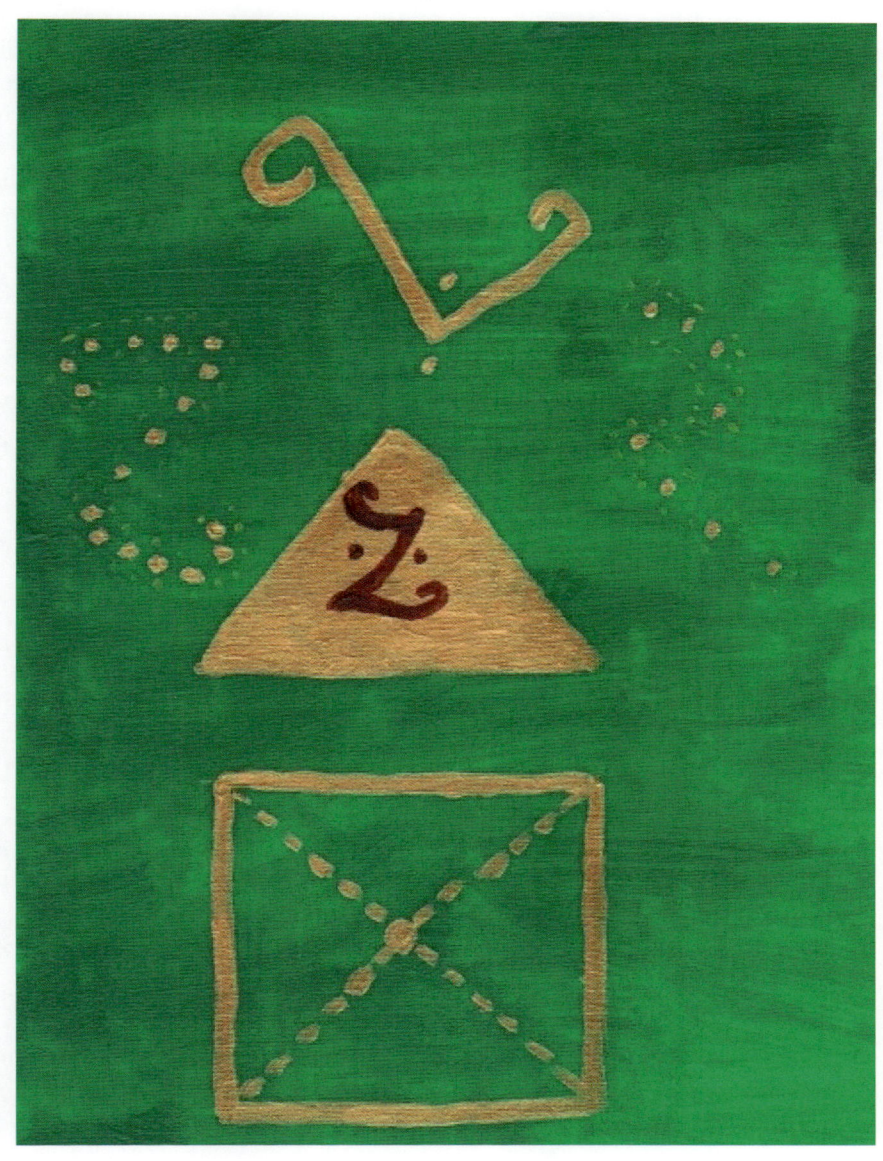

I was researching something in one of Diana Cooper's books and came across the Elemental Master Taia, All the book said was that Taia was the Elemental Master of earth. I knew it was unlikely that Diana was wrong but had to check with some friends as when I googled her name I didn't find anything about her. Interestingly, they couldn't find the reference to Taia in the book I had been reading. I was then given a message by one of my friends who said that Taia is from Merlin's book and that he wrote about this being of light and that there is a connection with Lady Gaia as well. I was then told that I was to connect with Taia through meditation in a quartz crystal pyramid.

Here is the information I gained from Taia during that meditation:

Taia : *'I am Taia I am the one that Merlin wrote about.*
We are to work together my child for there is a need for people to understand more about Mother Earth, about her healing needs and about those of us who are working with her.

You are aware of the beauty now within Mother Earth and such beauty it is but as you look through the beauty look beyond and what do you see?'

Me : 'I can see what looks like energy lines but they are not running smoothly they are zig zagged. It looks as if there's areas where there is energy pooling'

Taia: *'I am the keeper of these ley lines and those of us in Middle Earth are working hard to clear them so that the energies flow. Where there is pooling of energy is where there is episodes that you call Acts of God occur. This is because Mother Earth has to clear the negativity that is within those pools of energy.*

We need light workers to send light down into Middle Earth so that we can anchor it in where it is needed; we need assistance with clearing the ley lines.

I am also responsible for the crystal grids within Mother Earth for these connect with the crystal grids surrounding Mother Earth and they connect with the energies of the universe.'

Me: 'So Taia may I ask you is your role only to look after the ley lines and crystal grids within Mother Earth?'

Taia: *'There is far more to Middle Earth than you realise. Many are here who* have previously ascended and left the 3D world. They come here because they are in a higher dimension. We have beings of light here who are fifth, sixth and seventh dimension. We are all working to help Mother Earth and Lady Gaia to ascend.'

Me: 'May I ask what your relationship to Gaia is?'

Taia: *'I am Gaia's Twin Flame I am the masculine energies to her feminine energies.'*

Me: 'May I ask what your connection to Merlin is?'

Taia: *'Merlin is one of the guardians and great guides of the Earth. Merlin and I work closely together. Each of us has gifts that complement the other. We are twin souls but not twin flames.*

Merlin is seen as the great alchemist but he is one of many. I too have gifts that some would consider to be magic but it is how you define magic that is important. Many in your world associate the word magic with dark energies but magic can be used in the world of light too and indeed each of us has many gifts that we can work with to assist with the ascension process.

While scientists believe that Mother Earth is molten inside they do not understand that Mother Earth is a spiritual being and as such Middle Earth is a beautiful place to be.'

You were right about Merlin too and about Gaia for the three of us are linked the three of us work closely together. The three of us form a triangle; the three of us can form a pyramid, the three of us are very powerful together.

We wish to awaken many more souls on the Earth Plane. For as more souls awaken more light is drawn in to assist Mother Earth. There are many who have gifts that will help them on their path which will in turn help Mother Earth we wish to awaken these gifts through the channellings that you will receive from me and indeed from Gaia and Merlin.'

Me: 'I understood my work was to be with the angels. I promised to help them to bring a message of love and peace before I was born.'

Taia: *'Yes you must continue your work with the angels but we all work together* *for we are all one as you already know. We need your help we need your assistance. Earth is ascending and is ascending more quickly than ever expected but there is still much to be done and there are many down here in Middle Earth whom you on the Earth Plane need to know about. Those of you who are ready; those of you who are awakened; for you can connect with us and work with us to bring light to the core of the Earth. Much healing has begun but there is still a lot to be done. For man has spent eons living on Earth taking from her continually, not considering how she may be affected by the things he is doing. This cannot continue and it is important for us to work with those of you that are ready to assist Earth with her healing process.*

The crystal grids are in need of some work they need clearing and cleansing and then they will need to be realigned with the new energies on Earth. The energies are constantly changing and so the crystal grids must be aligned to meet these changing energies.

There are crystalline pyramids within Middle Earth each one has a significance. There are temples of healing in Middle Earth so that those of us that are here can keep our vibration high and clear our energy regularly.

There are beings on planet Earth who have left because of the damage done by man. Man talks about them as being extinct and indeed I suppose they are but in actual fact their vibration was higher and they left the planet. Some have gone elsewhere; others have come to Middle Earth to work from within.'

Me: 'Are you a wizard?'

Taia: *'I am an alchemist.'*

Me: 'What do you work with?'

Taia: *'I work with light and for light I work with love and for love, for I am love and light. I am one with Mother Earth and with the universe.'*

Me: 'You are an immense being to me.'

Taia: *'I am an Elemental Master. I am an Elemental Master of Earth not just the element earth but of Earth herself. I am an advisor to Earth. I too am a guardian of Earth. I am a guardian of Middle Earth I work with the energies of crystals within Middle Earth to assist with the cleansing process that needs to* *take place.'*

Me: 'What else do you work with?'

Taia: *'I have healing gifts that I am able to use within Middle Earth. Gaia and I work very closely together and we work with the galactic masters, angels and archangels and with source too.*

Everything that happens has precision, everyone works with precision, for we know exactly where the energies are to enter Earth and therefore where and how they will come to Middle Earth, but for now my child I have told you enough. We will meet again soon for there is much for me to tell you much for us to discuss. For I want to give you an understanding of Middle Earth as well as my role and how I work with Merlin and Gaia, but for now what you have is sufficient. Know that I am working closely with you with the book that you are currently writing and that I will work with you with other things as well that are connected to the Earth and the natural world. I know that you see the beauty of your planet I know that you love Mother Earth I know that everything that you do is with love.

Me: 'Thank you Taia.

Taia works closely with Archangel Gersia too, particularly with the energy grids and leylines. She has a beautiful energy and will work with you to bring more light into Mother Earth.

'I am Taia and it is with great love that I am with you today. There are many new energies currently coming into the Earth, that on the surface appear to be causing chaos. These energies are forcing people to heal and balance their karma so that they can hold more light.

Their Earth Star chakras are more open so that the higher vibration energies can be anchored into the Earth. As they allow themselves to heal we will open their Earth Star chakras further. Their Soul Star chakras are being opened too so that more light can come in through each and every being on the planet who is of light.

As the new energies are anchored into Middle Earth we are able to use them to clear the ley lines and support the energy grids. These energies too will assist us with clearing the pools of negativity that man has created, so that the effects of clearing them has less of an impact.

However there is still a need for some clearing which will cause changes within the Earth's crust which will lead to what you term as natural disasters. These are necessary not only to clear the energies but to balance the karma created by man.

More and more higher vibration energies will continue to enter the Earth plane and those of you who are ready will continue to lift your vibration. Each of you is helping us by healing yourselves and clearing your karma. We love and honour you and thank you for your assistance.'

Channelled by Sarah Hunt 15/11/14

THE EARTH'S CHAKRAS

It must be remembered that the Earth is a living, breathing organism with energy moving in and around her. Like all living things the Earth has main chakras (or main energy centres) in various places around her. She is also surrounded by an energetic body or aura, just the same as any other living being.

The Earth's chakras are connected by energy circuits known as ley lines which allow energy to run freely around the Earth and from one chakra to another. Earth also has many smaller chakras which connect many of the smaller ley lines that run through and around her.

There are many areas of the world where the Earth's energies are very strong.

Let's have a look at each chakra now.

The Root Chakra Mount Shasta California

The root chakra is located at Mount Shasta in northern California and is an extremely energetic site as it is home to one of the most massive volcano eruptions on earth. The Hupa, a northern California Indian tribe, has traditionally recognized Mt. Shasta as a sacred place and there are many stories of the mountains' powerful healing properties.

The Sacral Chakra Lake Titicaca, Bolivia/Peru

Lake Titicaca is home to the sacral chakra of the Earth. There are many mysteries associated with Lake Titicaca, the salty lake that once was adjacent to the sea. It was pushed up violently to its current location 12,000 feet in the Andes mountains in between modern day Peru and Bolivia just 10,000 years ago and legend associates this place with Atlantis.

Ley lines connect the chakra centers to each other and the one which joins the root chakra in Mount Shasta to this chakra is known as the Plumed Serpent.

The Solar Plexus Chakra   Uluru and Kata Tjuta, Austrailia

 Uluru rock, formerly known by its European name Ayers Rock, is the location of the Earth's solar plexus chakra. This place has always been known as a sacred place by the Aborigines.

The other great ley line, the Rainbow Serpent, emerges at Uluru from underground, and follows an energetic line to Katatjuta. Once in Katatjuta, which is a natural cathedral of sorts, it is shaped into various energies to be used by the many different species of life on Earth. It then exits through a heart shaped stone known as Ngunngarra, coming to the surface where it goes to Bali and intersects with the Plumed Serpent.

The Heart Chakra   Glastonbury and Shaftesbury

The Earth's heart chakra is located in one of the most famous holy places on Earth, marked by the centers known as Somerset, Shaftesbury, Dorset and Glastonbuy, in England.

Glastonbury Tor, an ancient sacred mound, has been called the "Heart of England" and is connected with numerous legends, going back through medieval times and continuing today.

The Throat Chakra   Great Pyramid, Mount Sinai, and Mount Olives (Middle East)

The throat chakra, exists in the area marked by the Great Pyramid, which is a monument erected in its honor. This chakra is unique because it does not exist on a ley line but on a spinning vortex of energy which is the voice of the Earth.

Geographically, this chakra is located in the exact centre of the Earth's landmass. It is a sacred area to many cultures and is home to ancient wisdom that is passed down, some say, from ancient Atlantis.

Interestingly it has been suggested that the modern day turmoil that exists in the Middle East is a physical manifestation of the cries of Mother Earth, who wants us to come to consciousness and awaken to our spiritual selves. The physical fracturing that is apparent in the turmoil being acted out in the Middle East is representative of the spiritual turmoil that has gripped mankind. By answering her call and allowing ourselves to awaken we can then learn to work with the energies in a positive way and in harmony with the Earth, so that we can be the limitless beings we were always intended to be.

The Third Eye Chakra   Western Europe

The third eye chakra moves each time that we enter a new age in order to facilitate the energy entering the earth during that age. This chakra opens portals and allows extra-dimensional energy to enter the Earth and is currently in Western Europe, which is the location of the major crop circle activity.

Crop circles are thought to be physical communication between Earth and Higher dimensions. When we enter the age of Capricorn in 2000 years' time the Third Eye chakra will reside near Recife, Brazil.

The Crown Chakra   Mount Kailas, Himalayas, Tibet

The crown chakra is located in Tibet. Its keepers, the people of Tibet have kept humanity's collective energy connected to the Earth's at this most holy of holy places for thousands of years. The people's highly developed level of consciousness partly comes from their close contact to this highly energetic place. This chakra emanates the True Will, the Earth's True Purpose.

Healing the Earth's Chakras

We can help to heal and balance the Earth's chakras by meditating on each of them and filling them with love. This may be done with assistance from any of the elementals.

Meditation

Make yourself comfortable and take a few deep breaths whilst putting your protection around you. Keep your focus on your breathing for the next few moments and allow your body and mind to completely relax.

Now become aware of being in a beautiful meadow. The sun is shining and there is a warm breeze blowing through your hair. Take in the beautiful energies of the countryside as you walk through the meadow.

As you look around you, you become aware of a beautiful unicorn coming towards you. Walk towards the unicorn and take a few moments to connect with the unicorn and ask it if you can work with it to help heal Mother Earth.

The unicorn tells you that together you can fill the Earth's chakras with love and asks you to get on its back as it is going to take you to each of the chakras.

As you make yourself comfortable on the unicorn's back you suddenly find yourself in the air. The unicorn tells you that it is taking you to the Earth's root chakra at Mount Shasta.

As you reach Mount Shasta the Unicorn asks you to open your crown and heart chakras and ask for the energies of unconditional love to flow through you and into the Earth's root chakra. As you do this you see a beautiful pink light coming from the universe down through your crown chakra and out of your heart chakra into the root chakra of the Earth. You watch the Earth's root chakra fill and balance itself with the help of the energies of love and then you see these energies moving out along the ley lines, clearing and cleansing them as it goes.

Once the unicorn is happy that the root chakra is cleansed and balanced you find yourself being taken to the sacral chakra in Lake Titicaca. As you arrive there you see the energies of love coming along the ley lines into the chakra and the unicorn asks you to open your crown and heart chakras again and send unconditional love into the sacral chakra to add to the energies moving into it. You watch the sacral chakra completely fill with the energies of love and then the energies move out into the ley lines cleansing and clearing them and filling them with love too.

Your unicorn then takes you to the solar plexus chakra in Uluru Australia. As you arrive there you see the chakra starting to fill with the energies of love which are coming along the ley lines and you find your crown and heart chakras opening as you send out more love from the universe into this chakra. You watch as the chakra fills and balances itself. The energies then once again move out into the ley lines clearing and balancing them as they go.

Your unicorn takes you to the Earth's heart centre in Glastonbury. As you reach Glastonbury you can see the energies of love coming along the ley lines into the Earth's heart centre. Once again you allow your crown and heart chakras to open so that you can send the unconditional love of the universe into the heart centre of the Earth. As you do this you become aware of the earth's heart centre opening and unconditional love flowing from it out into the universe.

The unicorn then takes you to the Earth's throat chakra at the Great Pyramid and as you arrive you can see the energies of love flow into the throat chakra. You open your crown and heart chakras and allow universal unconditional love to flow into the throat chakra and watch as the chakra fills and balances. As before the energies then move out into the ley line.

The unicorn moves off again and takes you to the Third Eye Chakra in Western Europe. You watch the energies of love moving along the ley lines into this chakra and open your crown and heart chakras so that you can send the universal energies of unconditional love into it. The chakra fills and balances with the energies of love.

The unicorn then takes you to the crown chakra at Mount Kalias in the Himalayas. As you arrive you are aware of the crown chakra already starting to fill with the energies of love and again you open your crown and heart chakras and send out universal unconditional love this time into the Earth's crown chakra.

As this chakra fills and balances the unicorn takes you up above the Earth and asks you to look down at the Earth. As you look you can see that the Earth is completely filled with love. The unicorn asks you to once again open your crown and heart chakras and send universal unconditional love to the Earth so that this time she is completely surrounded in love. As you watch you become aware of the Earth being completely surrounded in love so that her whole energy system is filled with love and you start to feel a sense of peace coming from her.

Feel yourself connect with the Earth as you surround her in love and connect with the peaceful feeling of the universe.

The unicorn thanks you for your help and tells you that it is now time for you to return to the meadow. He takes you back to the meadow and you thank him for his time and help. He tells you that he will be pleased to help you anytime you wish to help heal Mother Earth.

Now be aware of the images of the meadow starting to fade and start to bring yourself back to this time and space, grounding yourself before opening your eyes.

THE NEED FOR EARTH HEALING

Mother Earth has been abused by man over many thousands of years and this abuse goes back to the downfall of Atlantis. Man has forgotten that we are here to live in harmony with the Earth and all who reside on her and so there has been a lot of damage done to her.

Part of the healing process for Mother Earth has been through some major events which we call natural disasters. Natural disasters seem to me to happen for many reasons. Firstly as part of the healing process an area may need to be cleansed in some way, so with a Tsunami for example, the land is being cleansed with water. I was told in meditation, that the Tsunami in Japan was to clear the negativity from the nuclear bombs that had been tested in that area in previous years.

It is my understanding that the people who pass during such an event have agreed to do so to help to clear their own karma and the karma between man and the Earth.

These events also help to bring humans together so that they work with love and compassion for each other and with each other to help those who have lost everything or been hurt or lost loved ones.

Of course there is far more going on underneath all of this when these events happen as we are being shown that the most important thing is love and that love heals everything.

Whenever we are healing, whether it is on ourselves or others, or indeed whilst helping Mother Earth, the intention must come from the heart. Unconditional love is very important as love heals everything.

Forgiveness is also important and as we learn to heal ourselves we also need to learn to forgive all those who have hurt us and ourselves as well, for allowing them to do it.

When we help to heal Mother Earth it is important for us to forgive all those who have affected her, including ourselves. We also need to learn to give back to the Earth as well as take from her. She provides us with an abundance of ways and means for supporting ourselves and we need to remember to say thank you to her.

There are many little things that we can do on a day to day basis that will help reduce the number of resources that we use. For example, growing some of your own fruit and vegetables. You don't need a big garden to do this as most things can be grown in pots, but by doing this you are cutting down on the resources and packaging that is needed to supply some of your foods and even more importantly you are gaining an appreciation of the Earth, and the seasons and how they can affect what you are growing.

You could also walk to work or to the shop or your friend's house instead of taking the car. Whilst walking may take longer it will help to ground you with the Earth's energies. It will give you the opportunity to see the many things in nature that you would normally miss. It will enable you to experience the beautiful fragrances in the air on a warm summer evening. It will enable you to connect with yourself and your guides.

I am often given inspiration by my guides whilst walking to work and it gives me a chance to clear my mind of the busy chatter that can be incessant. In effect what I am doing is a walking meditation.

I am also connecting with nature once again which is something many of us, me included, don't do enough of. Connecting with nature will assist you with connecting with these beautiful beings of light from the Nature and Elemental Kingdoms so that you can strengthen your connection with them and work with them to heal yourself and Mother Earth.

We all have a need to connect with ourselves on a much deeper level and to let go of the ego self. We need to learn to listen to our very essence the part of us that knows what is for our highest good. We need to learn to love ourselves for we cannot truly love others unless we love ourselves. Loving ourselves unconditionally is important because we do not know the bigger picture, at times all we see are some of the jigsaw pieces. It is only when we look back that we can start to see the bigger picture.

We are all on Earth at this time because we have agreed to be here. We all have karmic debt that needs to be addressed and balanced. Some of it may be thousands of years old. We are here to assist Mother Earth with the ascension process and we can do this in many ways but one of the most important things that we can do is learn to heal ourselves and connect with ourselves.

My Reiki students know that what I constantly bang on about is self-healing! In my opinion it is the most important thing you can do because the world around you is a mirror of what is happening inside. So when you have chaos ensuing around you it is an indication of chaos going on inside.

When you are surrounded by clutter then there is clutter inside. When you have had a clear out in your house it is an indication that you are letting go of thoughts and emotions that no longer serve you.

When you allow yourself to heal, when you allow yourself to forgive, you start to allow unconditional love to flow. When you learn to love unconditionally you are not condoning the behaviour of others, you are freeing yourself and them from the negativity that you would otherwise get caught up in by judging them and yourself. When you learn to love yourself unconditionally you can then truly love others.

When you take responsibility for your healing and your thoughts, words and actions you are able to step into the flow of your life and bring more positive people and experiences into it. You cannot heal others including the Earth, effectively if you are not willing to look at yourself.

I have had a simple message on many occasions when I have been going through difficult times. The words 'Healer heal thyself' always pop into my mind. It's a reminder to me to work on myself first because I cannot change anyone, I can only change myself. I am not in control of anyone, I am only in control of myself.

If you want the world to be a peaceful, loving place, then you must find that peaceful, loving place within you first. When you have found it within you, you will find it around you as you will draw others in who are loving and peaceful people. The more of us that do this and hold a vision of love and peace on the Earth, the quicker we will be able to make Earth a planet filled with peace and love.

As we learn to heal ourselves we are able to hold more light in our energy systems, so we are able to shine more light out into the world and indeed the universe. Light will penetrate even the darkest of corners. The more of us that are willing to heal ourselves, the more light we will hold. As we hold more light it will shine out to Mother Earth. As we heal and learn to love unconditionally those energies of love will move between us, the universe and Mother Earth.

The Nature Angels, Elemental Masters and elemental beings are waiting to work with you to help you to heal yourself as well as Mother Earth. Are you ready to work with them to create the life of love and peace that your soul craves?

A LIGHTWORKERS PRAYER

I was on my way to a Mind Body Soul show in Corby when these words started to come to me. I asked the angels to wait until I could write them down as they felt important to share. So here they are as a reminder of how we can bring more peace and love into the world.

'Angels of light keep me safe,

Angels of light surround me in your love,

Angels of light fill me with your light,

Angels of light empower me to be my true self,

Angels of light I love you,

Angels of light open my heart,

Angels of light help me to be a beacon for those who need my help,

Angels of light surround me in your love for I am a child of the universe,

Angels of light help me to bring your message of peace and love to the world.

Thank you '

Channelled from the Angelic Realm 15.11.14

May your life be filled with peace and love as you help to heal the Earth.

Sarah

BIBLIOGRAPHY

Nature Spirits and Elemental Beings   Marko Pogacnik

Nature Spirits The Remembrance   Susan Raven

http://www.crystalinks.com/grids.html

http://www.childrenofthesun.org/index.php?option=com_content&view=article&id=49&Itemid=54

http://hiddenlighthouse.wordpress.com/category/earth-grid/

http://www.bibliotecapleyades.net/mapas_ocultotierra/esp_mapa_ocultotierra_10.htm

http://crystl37.blogspot.co.uk/2011/04/mainstream-science-discovers.html

A New Light on Angels   Diana Cooper

ABOUT THE AUTHOR

Sarah Hunt is a Reiki Master Teacher attuned to several systems of Reiki, although her main focus is Usui/Tibetan Reiki which she teaches to all levels. Sarah is also a Past Life Regression Therapist, Spiritual Medium, Divine Channel for the Archangels, Psychic Artist and Spiritual Teacher.

Sarah connected with the Angelic Realm in 2011 after being given a message from Archangel Gabriel at a crystal workshop she was running. She was told that it was time to fulfill a promise she had made to the angels before she was bring to help to bring their message of peace and love to the world. She started working with the Nature Angels in 2012 and then with the Elemental Masters. Whilst writing this book she connected with a new Elemental Master whom she has introduced here, but whom Sarah knows she will be working with for some time, which will enable her to bring more information to you all in the future about Earth healing.

Sarah also offers Reiki treatments and workshops, Past Life Regression Therapy, Meditation, Crystal and Angel workshops, Angel Attunements, readings and paints healing energy pictures channelled from the Angelic Realm. She also accepts commissions for paintings which will have the healing energies that you need emitted from the picture.

For more information about Sarah and her work please go to :

www.peaceful-living.co.uk

Other books written by Sarah include:

Reiki A Pathway to Self
ISBN 978-1475101942

Meditation: A Beginners Guide
ISBN 978-1502828439

Healing Mandalas and Messages from the Angels of Atlantis
ISBN 978-1502891822

As a 'Thank You' for purchasing my book the following items which complement this book are available to you from my website www.peaceful-living.co.uk at discounted prices.

Earth Healing with the Nature Angels & Elemental Masters Meditation CD's.

Normally £11.49 including p&p. Use the following code when you order and get the CD set for £10.00 incl p&p. **Discount Voucher Code:** 14ehm5jb

Printed in Great Britain
by Amazon